HEALING

with

COLOR & LIGHT

HEALING
— *with* —
COLOR & LIGHT

THEO GIMBEL
with Gaia Books

A GAIA ORIGINAL

A Fireside Book
Published by Simon & Schulster Inc.

New York London Toronto Sydney Tokyo Singapore

A GAIA ORIGINAL

Conceived by   Joss Pearson

Editorial   Eleanor Lines

Design and Illustration   Lucy Guenot

Direction   Joss Pearson
Patrick Nugent

FIRESIDE
Rockefeller Center
1230 Avenue of the Americas
New York, New York 10020

Copyright © 1994 Gaia Books Ltd, London

Typeset by Select Typesetters, London
Reproduction by Global Colour, Malaysia
Printed and bound in Hong Kong by Mandarin Offset

10   9   8   7   6   5   4   3   2   1

Library of Congress Cataloging in Publication Data

Gimbel, Theo.
   Healing with color and light: improve your mental, physical,
   and spiritual health/by Theo Gimbel.
      p.   cm.
   "A Fireside book".
   ISBN 0-671-86857-8
   1. Color – Therapeutic use. I. Title.
RZ414.6.G55   1994
615.8'31 – dc 20

93-31072
CIP

ISBN: 0-671-86857-8

how to use this book

This book presents a comprehensive summary of the scientific basis of color therapy, of the treatments and techniques used, and of how to treat with color. There are also exercises and practical activities, indicated by a solid bar above the text. By following the instructions you can begin your therapeutic work in color at home.

The book can be used on its own or in conjunction with a professional training in color therapy. For a professional qualification you will require a personal tutor (see Resources, p. 124).

For diagnosis and treatment of serious illness, you should always consult a qualified color practitioner. Under the professional code of practice for color practitioners, all color therapy treatments for serious illness should be given under medical supervision. Color therapy can be used successfully in conjunction with Western medicine.

foreword

Theo Gimbel's work in color therapy is both stimulating and challenging. This important book opens new doors to the possibilities of holistic healing, incorporating the 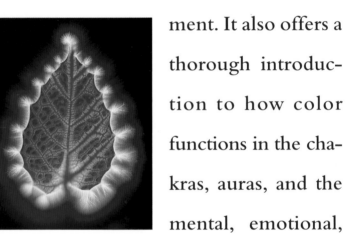 powerful and ever-present world of color into other therapeutic methods such as relaxation, meditation, visualization, breathing, and movement. It also offers a thorough introduction to how color functions in the chakras, auras, and the mental, emotional, metabolic, and physical dimensions of health. With over 25 years of experience, Gimbel presents an approach that will appeal to many readers seeking to better understand the interconnectedness of all life and the role that color plays in maintaining health and wellbeing. He presents simple but effective exercises and practices that can be used with friends or individually, as well as more advanced methods of diagnosis and treatment that require professional color practitioners. Simply reading this book will expand our understanding of color and light. By practicing Gimbel's exercises and techniques, we can move along the healing path that leads to an enriched awareness of the world – and the human body – in all its beauty and color.

CONTENTS

introduction

Color is an experience. It is one that we, on this planet, are uniquely privileged to enjoy.

The spectrum of electromagnetic energies that emanate from the sun and irradiate the Earth includes the range that we "see" as light. The varying wavelengths of this energy are reflected back to our eyes from the objects they strike and interpreted by our brains as the various hues of the color spectrum, so that when we view the world in terms of color, in fact, the color is in our minds, not in the landscape. As John Stewart Collis says in *The Vision of Glory:*

> *"We see the yellow daffodil growing up out of the ground, and it seems clear that its color, the most emphatic thing about it, grows up with it, belongs to it. Yet no; that yellow on the daffodil, that red on the rose was eight minutes ago in the sun.*

This manifestation of color results from a very fine balance of factors: the receptive abilities of our eyes and brain, and the combination of gases, moisture, and dust particles in the Earth's atmosphere that filter, reflect, and refract the rays of light energy. Without this atmosphere there would be no life on Earth and little color. Too many particles in the atmosphere, either from

natural causes or industrial pollution, can create a blanket that some of the light rays cannot penetrate. When the light level is reduced in this way, or when it declines gradually at dusk, the color experience fades and we are left in a world of monotones.

None of us see color in quite the same way, or to the same intensity. We tend to think of it as a purely physical phenomenon experienced by our sense of sight alone, but as a form of energy, color is active at all levels of our being – mental, emotional, physical, and spiritual. Hence its effects are not restricted only to the sighted. Those with impaired vision are equally receptive to these energies, and in many cases are more so because of their enhanced sensitivity to non-visual stimuli.

As you work through this book, you will discover that each color has its individual characteristics and effects. Some of these you may use intuitively in your dress and make-up to reveal or disguise your true feelings and intentions; some will already be familiar to you as everyday cliches used to express emotions and feelings: "red with anger", "green with envy". Extremes of emotions are often the outward display of imbalances or blockages in the flow of color energies into and out of the body. Analysis of these imbalances can reveal ailments before they manifest in the physical body, and color therapy treatments, such as controlled exposure to colored light, can adjust and correct the energy flow.

The later chapters of this book describe techniques of color diagnosis such as perceiving and interpreting the colored aura that surrounds all living things, and using a pendulum to dowse the color energies in the vertebrae of the spine. There are charts to aid the analysis and diagnosis of illness, and the choice of suitable treatments. Some of these are straightforward enough for you to work at on your own: a change of color scheme in your home or workplace may be all that is needed. In some cases more advanced techniques may be called for, such as the use of crystals or colored light. These will require the guidance of a trained practitioner.

The exercises in this book, in particular the breathing, visualization, and meditation exercises, will enable you to raise your color perception and fine-tune your senses to open yourself up to the healing color energies. You will enjoy the benefits of this active approach to color at all levels of your being – physical, mental, emotional and, most importantly, spiritual.

Without life there is little color; without color there is no life.

CHAPTER ONE

color in our world

The importance of color

We are bathed in color all our lives, even from the moment of conception: light penetrates translucent skin and muscle to envelop the developing fetus in a reddish-golden glow. Born into a world of colors, we grow surrounded by color in the environment and in our homes; we dress in colorful clothes, eat colorful foods, and make choices that are informed by color every day. Rarely if at all do we have a colorless experience: a white space without form, or complete darkness. Instead, through the changing contrast of dark and light we perceive the colors in our human world and our surroundings.

Color dominates our senses. We learn at an early age to interpret our environment as much by color as by shapes or sounds. Our response to color is so basic that, until the age of about five, six, or even later, children who are asked to sort colored shapes automatically divide them according to their color, rather than their shape. Boys and girls develop in slightly different ways: whereas girls maintain their level of response to color, boys start to respond more to shape at an earlier age.

Throughout life we continue to use color as a cue for interpreting what we see: grey hair tells us of middle age; grey landscapes speak of cities; a red apple tells of its ripeness; red traffic lights bring us to a halt. Color coding guides our travels, our administration, and such practical details as electric wiring. Color gives us information about much of our environment; it even helps us to locate ourselves geographically, by the hue of the local stone, for example, or the tones of the colors in a landscape.

Color messages

At another level, we make statements about our mood with the colors we wear, and we can read how our friends feel, too, through their color statements. The colors we see around us can noticeably affect our states of mind and our feelings – the color in a red room produces very different sensations from those in a room painted blue. Color schemes alter the amount and the type of light that our eyes, our skin, and even the underlying tissues and organs receive. And color is strongly linked with emotions. By describing

Darkness and light

The Bible says, "In the beginning God created the heaven and the earth.

And the earth was without form, and void; and darkness was upon the face of the deep. And the spirit of God moved upon the face of the waters.

And God said, Let there be light: and there was light."

Genesis 1:1

The energy of light came out of darkness: darkness pervaded the world before light appeared. We need both light and darkness in our lives, just as seeds need both darkness and light to germinate.

God sleeps in the stone
God dreams in the plant
God moves in the animal
God awakes in man

*Translated from Ancient
Chinese wisdom*

people as "green with envy", "purple with rage", "yellow with cowardice", or "seeing red", we are using common color associations that may have more truth than we realize.

Such associations are only part of our lifelong relationship with color: we live by the rhythm of color changes that denote the passage of time and the cycle of seasons. As day passes, the daylight colors change and are infinitely mobile in their hues. The deep blue of the sky before dawn gives way to the paler blue light that permeates mornings; this is followed by the more yellow hue of the afternoon and then the red light of the evening. These shifts can be so gradual that they are hardly noticeable, but nonetheless they color our perception of the passing day (see right). The seasons, too, highlight very different colors, with the fresh greens of spring darkening as the summer progresses, and providing

Color and photography

You can experiment with your camera to see how colors change during the course of a clear day. Find a place where you can take pictures of green grass, blue sky, and some red or orange objects, such as flowers, in the early morning, mid-morning, at mid-day, in the mid-afternoon, and in the early evening.

a blaze of orange, yellow, and gold only a few months later. Winter introduces a stark note, with few vivid colors, and sometimes a smattering of snow that obliterates the remaining green, reducing the outlook to a simple contrast between darkness and light. Many of us live in houses that offer light at any time of the day and night, and heat or coolness throughout the year, and so to some extent we lose contact with the natural rhythms of the daily and yearly cycles.

Responding to the invisible

In addition to visible light the sun emits high-energy cosmic rays, gamma rays, X-rays, and ultra-violet, which have a subtle impact on us all the time. The Earth's atmosphere, in particular the ozone layer, protects us from much of their harmful effects. Little is documented about the way in which this background radiation affects us.

Light as visible energy

Our eyes translate the energy of light into signals – nervous impulses – that the brain interprets as "seeing". This visible light is part of a wider spectrum of energy that surrounds us (see p. 34), and most of this comes from the sun. Visible light is made up of the colors that we know as the rainbow. Our eyes are sensitive to the whole range of its hues, but the rest of the spectrum is invisible to us. Although these energies, such as infrared and ultraviolet, are outside our conscious color vision, we are nonetheless sensitive to them to some extent (see left).

Light and its constituent colors have a strong effect on both mind and body. At physical, mental, and emotional levels we respond to colors whether we realize it or not.

Physical responses to color

As a general rule, the red end of the spectrum tends to make the body tense, while the blue end of the spectrum tends to relax it. Exposure to red increases the blood pressure, while blue relaxes the body and lowers blood pressure (see p. 20).

Mental responses to color

Color affects our perceptions. A red room seems smaller than a blue one, for example.

Emotional responses to color

Color affects the way we feel about what we see. This is connected to the physical responses and psychological associations developed from infancy onward. But in general, red excites us, while blue makes us feel more calm.

Color and physiology

Color not only fills our outside world; it penetrates deep into our bodies. Its continual influence means that the effects of light on the body are second only to the effects of food.

The stained-glass window from Chartres Cathedral in France (right), transforms daylight into colors rich in spiritual overtones. The craft of creating stained glass, which reached its height in Europe during the 12th and 13th centuries, relies heavily on the ability of metallic oxides to "hold" the light and generate an atmosphere suitable for meditation and prayer.

Experiments on plants, which need light in order to make carbohydrates, show that exposing them only to red or green light, for example, radically alters the quality of their growth. When mustard and cress seeds were exposed to only red light, the developing plants were stunted with small foliage, and had a bitter taste. Exposure to only green light produced weak plants. In contrast, under blue light the seeds produced beautiful, well developed plants, which grew quite slowly, and had a very sweet flavour.

Of all the colors, red and blue light have the most marked effect on the physiology of the human body. Red light increases muscular activity, blood pressure, respiration, and heart rate. Blue has the opposite effect, relaxing the body, and can help insomnia sufferers (see also p. 101).

The pathways of light

Light energy received by the eye sets up nervous impulses on the retina, which travel as coded messages along the optic nerve to the visual cortex at the back of the brain. En route, some of these excitations trigger a specific part of the brain's hypothalamus, which acts as the body's biological clock by regulating sleeping, feeding, and other functions such as temperature and water balance.

The hypothalamus influences both the pituitary and pineal glands in the brain. These glands also respond to messages from all the body cells about the quantity and color quality of light shining on the body.

The pituitary and pineal glands conduct the functions of the body by producing hormones that stimulate other glands, such as the adrenals and reproductive organs, and affect the metabolism of the body.

The effect of color on our bodies does not depend on our eyesight alone. The superficial layers of skin and flesh – and even the skull – are particularly sensitive to ultraviolet light. Exposure to blue light over the whole body has long been a cure for children with jaundice, and ultraviolet light causes the skin to produce melanin (which gives us a tan) and vitamin D (which is crucial for the body's metabolism of calcium). In Russia, schoolchildren exposed to a supplement of invisible ultraviolet light apparently grew faster, had fewer colds, and produced better work. Experiments have shown that visually impaired people are affected by color in the same way as the sighted. Some are sensitive enough to identify a color with great accuracy by feeling the density of the air that surrounds it. The air over a red surface, for example, feels more dense than the air next to blue.

Incoming information from the visible and invisible parts of the spectrum is integrated and taken to every cell in the body (see left). This mechanism helps to orchestrate and harmonize our inner selves with the universe outside.

Too much or too little light can upset general health and wellbeing. People who are exposed to insufficient light, either because they spend too much time indoors in artificial light, which does not provide the full spectrum found in natural daylight energy (see Chapter Two), or because they live in latitudes where the sun is absent for long periods during the winter, are known to be prone to winter-time depression (see p. 37). By contrast, excessive exposure to light has been shown to speed development, and even have an ageing effect. For example, girls who live in towns and cities where the night is kept artificially light by high levels of street lighting, begin menstruation earlier than girls from more rural areas, who experience a normal day/night rhythm of light and darkness.

History of Color

Egypt

The ancient Egyptians listed on a papyrus from 1550BC a number of colored cures, including red lead, black lizards, and verdigris, a green copper salt which, when mixed with beetle wax, was used to treat cataracts. The Egyptians are said to have built temples where color healing took place. Sunlight shone through colored gems, such as rubies and sapphires, on to people seeking healing. They also used pulverized gemstones as remedies for sickness – yellow beryls, for example, as a cure for jaundice.

China

The Chinese have always diagnosed illness by reading the "color" of pulses, complexion, and the appearance of the body's tissues and organs. A red pulse indicates numbness of the heart, whereas a yellow pulse means the stomach is healthy. The *Nei Ching,* a medical text compiled almost 2000 years ago, records color diagnoses. "When the viscera are green like kingfishers' wings they are filled with life." On the other hand, "When their color is green like grass they are without life."

Europe

Color was also vital to the doctrine of the Four Humours. This system of medical thought may have originated in Egypt and was common throughout Europe from the days of the ancient Greeks and Romans to the Renaissance. Each humour was assigned its own color – red blood, black bile, yellow bile, and white phlegm. Any imbalance in the humours was manifested in the color of the skin complexion, tongue, urine, and faeces.

Correcting imbalances

Color practitioners can correct imbalances of energy inside the body using a variety of techniques that have been tried and tested over the last hundred years or more. The techniques include the use of full-spectrum lamps, colored crystals, silks, and shapes; wearing colored clothes, drinking solarized water, eating colorful foods, and the application of colored oils during massage (see Chapter Six). In addition, the techniques of color visualization, color breathing, and the use of movement enhance the effects of color (see Chapter Three). A color practitioner may receive training in any or all of these techniques. The use of full-spectrum lamps in healing is probably the most powerful of the techniques available to the color practitioner.

Color in make-up and clothes

For most of us, our awareness of color begins and ends with our clothes (and, for some of us, our make-up), and the colors of the rooms that surround us at home, at work, or in places we visit.

Our choice of clothes reflects the way we feel; the colors can also contribute to a healing process (see p. 105). Cosmetic psychologists claim that a woman can feel better about herself by adding particular colors to her face, and so begin a cycle of wellbeing. Real confidence, of course, springs from within and a naturally glowing face is the result of good health and diet, as well as happiness and wellbeing – the inner harmony on which color practitioners work.

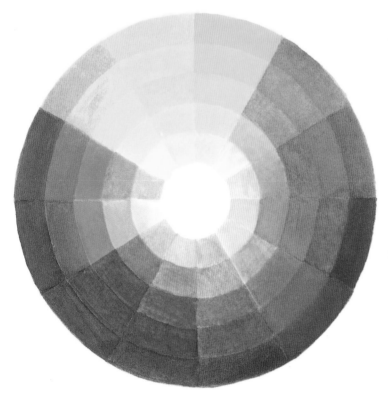

The Itten color wheel
Johannes Itten's work at the Bauhaus School led him to develop a graphic device that would enable artists to visualize the result of mixing colors (left).

Primary pigment colors are mixed to produce secondaries. For example, the primaries yellow and red make orange, a secondary color. Mixing orange and yellow produces orangey-yellow, a tertiary color. Itten's wheel demonstrated how adding black and white affected each color; the importance of this came from Itten's observations that colors appeared harmonious if, together, they yielded a neutral shade of grey.

Cosmetic colors can appear to alter the dimensions of your face by changing the color of your hair, skin, lips, and eye make-up. This may make you feel better about yourself but there is no substitute for the natural face (right), which glows with the spirit of inner wellbeing.

Color therapy works on this inner harmony. While the superficial applications of colored fabrics and oils enhance the work of the practitioner, they cannot be as effective as a complete color treatment using full-spectrum colored lights.

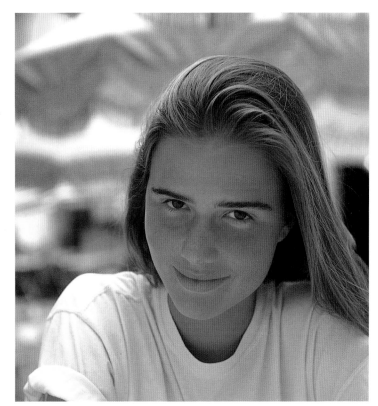

The origin of cosmetic advice

In an attempt to represent the relationships between colors, and to indicate how one color affects the appearance of another, Johannes Itten, a lecturer at the Bauhaus School in Germany in the 1920s, developed his color wheel. Itten expressed colors not only in terms of hue, but in their "cold" or "warm" appearance. Yellow, yellow-orange, orange, red, and red-violet are warm, while yellow-green, green, blue, blue-violet, and violet are cold. The intermediate hues may appear to be more or less warm or cold, depending on their adjacent colors.

Itten was fascinated by designs, and the connections between color, form, and music. He also noted that his students' color choices complemented the colors of their skin, hair, and eyes. His observations gave rise to skin color analysis tests, which formed the basis for a most successful cosmetic consultancy service.

Color at school

For a young child of 6 to 7 years, the color rose pink enhances the child's emotional as well as active involvement in the class. In the Waldorf school in Göttingen, Germany (below), the color scheme for each year's classroom is subtly different, moving toward yellow for 12 year olds. This reflects their increasing mental activity. For the following year, a gentle green fills the classroom, allowing the teenagers to balance their thoughts and make careful judgements.

Color in the home and at work

For thousands of years the number of pigments available for coloring objects was limited. Artists, dyers, glaziers, and other crafts people used pigments such as woad, madder, cochineal, and Tyrian purple, derived from natural sources. The advent of artificial dyes in the latter half of the 19th century led to an explosion of color that continues to this day. Using modern techniques, small adjustments in the amount of black or white pigment added to the basic colors of the spectrum can create a myriad different tints or shades.

With the wealth of colors now available, information on the particular effects of different colors is now in demand. Color practitioners can advise on color use in the home, in hospitals and schools, and in offices and factories.

STAGE (blue)

HANDICRAFTS (orange/red)

KITCHEN (yellow)

CLASS 7 (yellow/green)

HALL (pale red/pink)

CLASS 8 (pale green)

DINING ROOM (orange/yellow)

FOYER (red)

EURYTHMY 1 (pale pink)

CLASS 6 (orange/yellow)

CLASS 5 (pale orange)

CLASS 4 (pale orange)

EURYTHMY 2 (pale red)

CLASS 3 (orange/red)

CLASS 2 (pink/orange)

CLASS 1 (pink/red)

Each room in a home can be colored for a specific purpose. Take your cue from the warm and cool colors (see the Itten color wheel, p. 22). Use warm colors to stimulate activity in a room; use cool colors to produce a calming effect. Turquoise, for example, is a good color for a kitchen. It gives a fresh appearance and promotes calm activity. Use bright colors to promote alertness and highlight the parts of the kitchen that are potentially hazardous. Bedrooms need relaxing blues or greens, whereas the color of a study can tend toward more stimulating shades such as reds or browns, depending on the mood that the work requires. Greens and peachy-orange colors create a peaceful place to digest food and enjoy the company of friends (see the summary chart on pages 28-9).

Rudolf Steiner (1861-1925) studied the effects of color on individuals and developed a theory from which he produced color schemes for school rooms. His first school opened in Stuttgart in 1919. Steiner, known for his philosophical lectures and his work in education, considered that the most important aspect of a child's learning came directly from the developing spirituality. The scheme of colors that Steiner recommended for each age group is intended to reflect the child's stage of development (see facing page).

Hospital color schemes can help the healing process. Specially chosen colors in hospitals for the mentally ill have had dramatic effects. The following key words offer a useful basic guidance. They apply to all color schemes (see pp. 28-9), but have particular relevance for the healing needs of hospitals. Use red to increase energy; orange for joy; yellow for detachment; green to create balance; turquoise for immunity; blue for calmness; violet for dignity, and magenta to help bring about change.

Using these guidelines, blue may well predominate in a hospital for disturbed patients. Use violet at the patients' entrance to give a sense of dignity; orange at the staff entrance to begin the day in a cheerful way. Individual bedrooms can reflect a patient's needs: a lethargic patient, for example, would benefit from a rose-colored room; use turquoise for those of a nervous disposition, and blue for a restless patient.

The color of packaging
Psychologist Dr Max Lüscher
(see p. 97) put forward the idea
that the color of a product's
packaging in some way corresponds to the need that the product
fulfils. Products packaged in dark
blue, for example, offer security,
while someone who chooses a
product because of its yellowish-
red packaging is revealing a desire
to achieve and win.

In offices, factories, and other workplaces the management
of color is used to improve the working environment in
order to increase productivity and efficiency. More companies and organizations are making color an integral part
of a building's structure.

Green helps staff tolerate a noisy environment, blue is
good for cooling down a hot workplace, and occasional
architectural features painted red keep people moving.
However, too much of a color can have a different effect
from the one intended – excess red brings out aggression,
for example, while too much green makes staff over-relaxed.
Safety features, likewise, are based on the effects of exposure
to particular colors. Firefighting equipment, for example,
is colored red, as are signs indicating "stop", "don't", or
"danger". Green is commonly used to denote an "escape
route" or emergency exit.

Commercial products

Companies study and make use of our color associations
and preferences in order to sell us their products. Packaging
of products relies heavily on color, both to carry
information and to make the product attractive. Sugar, for
example, is sold in packets colored in bluey-pinks and blue
because, unlike green, these colors are associated with
sweetness. In experiments with washing powders, the
color of the packet has been shown to have a profound
influence on choice. Even though the powder in three
sample packets – colored yellow, blue, and yellow-blue –
was the same, customers thought the powder in the yellow
packet was too strong, that in the blue packet too weak. The
powder of choice was contained in the yellow-blue packet.
In similar research, coffee in a brown can was thought to be
too strong and in a red can too rich, in a blue can too mild
and in a yellow can too weak – even though the coffee was
the same in each case.

Fast-food outlets are often decorated with reds, yellows,
and whites. Red makes the place warm and inviting, but
also exciting so that it speeds the throughput of people.
Yellow together with white emphasises hygiene. The
combination creates a place where customers can relax and
enjoy their food but do not linger too long.

*The warm orange tones used in the
color scheme in this dining room
(right) enhance the pleasure of
entertaining friends for a meal.*

Summary of color effects

The chart on these two pages, based on the work of color practitioners, indicates the effects of the predominant colors in a room. It will help you to analyse your current interior color schemes as well as to plan any new ones. The details given in these guidelines apply to colors seen in daylight, or when full-spectrum lighting (see pp. 36-7) illuminates the room. Ordinary tungsten bulbs tend to add a yellowy-red appearance to the colors. Cool white fluorescent lighting also distorts colors, making them seem more blue.

Color	Room	Use/Effect
RED	Use in activity areas, passages Not bedrooms, offices, factories, stress areas	Makes rooms look smaller Increases pulse rate Stimulates inhalation Keeps us alert Facilitates judgement Enhances activity Oppressive and tiring when dense and strong
ORANGE	Suitable for dining areas, entertainment areas, dancing halls, passages Not bedrooms, study, or stress areas	Stimulates and enhances dance and movement Encourages joyfulness, lightness, release, pleasure
YELLOW	Pure yellow is difficult to use; best in rooms to be used alone Not in offices, bedrooms, study, or work areas	Encourages detachment, nervousness and shallow breathing Suits mature minds
GREEN	For places that need balanced judgement, including operating theatres Not most living areas or activity areas	Promotes balance and careful judgement Makes rooms look flat, dead and empty Encourages indecision Arrests movement, encourages stasis
TURQUOISE	Kitchen, bathroom, bedrooms, offices, treatment rooms Not activity and play areas	Cool, refreshing, calming, soothing Good for nervous inflammation

Pale colors, often used in homes, have the same type of effect as their more colorful counterparts. The addition of white, however, tones down the impact. For example, strong blue will relax you almost to the point of sleep, while a pale blue is mildly relaxing; a strong red is overstimulating and therefore tiring, while pink is mildly stimulating and increases alertness.

Remember that paints are rarely pure in color. Colors are mixed together and carry subtle tones that are not immediately apparent, but which nonetheless alter their effects.

Color	Room	Use/Effect
BLUE	Bedrooms, offices, treatment rooms, stress areas Not dining rooms or entertainment areas	Calms, relaxes, creates feeling of breathing out, and sleep Helps to combat tension, asthmatic conditions, nervousness, and insomnia
VIOLET	Where dignity is necessary – entrance halls to hospitals, places of worship and dedication, also festive areas, lecture rooms Not in wards, or treatment rooms	Encourages purpose, prayer and meditation For dignity, reverance Calms body and balances mind
MAGENTA	Chapels, entrance halls, lecture rooms Not in entertainment areas	Color of spiritual fulfilment Induces contentment, feeling of completeness, and self-respect
BLACK	Not suitable as an overall color	Heightens emotional response
WHITE	A stark color needing compensation with ornaments, paintings, plants, etc	Exaggerates purity Suggests a non-experience Gives stark effect

CHAPTER TWO

the science of color

The immediate effects of the color that surrounds you, both at home and at work, are easy to identify and use (see Chapter One). But a deeper understanding of the influence of color and how color can be used in therapy requires a closer look at how light brings color into the body, and how the body registers color messages.

How light enters the body

Our eyes are the most highly tuned of our organs for receiving colored light. They supply about 90 per cent of the sensory information available to the brain. But information about light and color also enters the body through the skin covering the whole surface of the body (see p. 20). Our eyes gather visual information, and channel it through to the brain so that we can perceive more accurately in consciousness what the body also experiences but does not make conscious (see pp. 48-9).

The physiology of light and color detection via the eyes is well established (see *The pathways of light,* p. 20). Light passes through the lens at the front of each eye and registers on the retina at the back. Within the retina, specialized cells, known as cones, respond to the whole color range, and these cells are at their most active during the day. As evening falls, a different set of light-sensitive cells, the rods, dominate vision. Although rods respond most readily to blue-green light they are sensitive to the intensity of light, whatever the color. Rods are responsible for night vision. The rod and cone cells convert the light that enters the eye into electrical impulses, which the optic nerve then conveys to the back of the brain for interpretation.

Color blindness

Some people are unable to register the difference between certain colors. Usually the difficulty is in distinguishing red from green, although other people cannot tell blue from yellow. About 8 per cent of men, and 1 per cent of women are red-green color blind. But conscious sensitivity to certain colors bears no relation to the physiological effects of those wavelengths. Even when red and green are both seen as a muddy brown, each color will have its different, specific effects on the body. As with visually impaired people, the impact of color does not depend on being able to see. Perceptions of color and light enter the body via the skin, even when clothed. All but the densest, darkest clothes allow light to penetrate. In this way, the predominant colors in the surroundings can still have their effect over the whole of the body.

History of color science

Pythagoras, Plato, and Aristotle developed some of the early theories about light and sight. Pythagoras (c582 – c507BC) believed that objects themselves gave off particles that made them visible. Plato (427–347BC) thought that the eye emitted light, which bounced off objects, giving information on their shape, color, and size. Aristotle (384–322BC) studied how light travels. His contribution was a theory that light travels in waves rather than particles. Aristotle's wave theory remains nearest to current thinking, but the wave versus particle argument raged for the next 2000 years, until physicists such as Max Planck (1858 – 1947) and Albert Einstein (1879 – 1955) laid the foundations for the currently accepted theory in the early years of the 20th century. Known as the "quantum" theory, it accepts elements of both the particle and the wave theories: light energy moves in discrete "packages", known as photons, and this movement may assume a wave form.

Isaac Newton (1642–1727) discovered that sunlight, although it appears to be white, is really a blend of colors. He performed a series of experiments in which he guided a shaft of sunlight through a glass prism in a darkened room so that the white light separated into its seven constituent colors – the colors of the rainbow.

Newton was a mathematician and philosopher before specializing in the science of optics, but like many men in the 17th century who were making discoveries at the forefront of science, he had a mystical side to his nature. He perceived seven colors in the spectrum (and seven is a mystical number). Goethe (1749 – 1832) identified six colors in the spectrum: three primary colors – red, yellow, blue – and three secondaries – orange, green, violet – the products of mixing the primaries. Goethe's reasoning came as much from his career as an artist as anything else: six colors served his practical purpose of mixing colors on a palette.

Wave energy

Electromagnetic waves have three features – wavelength, frequency (see p. 34), and amplitude. A wave with a short wavelength, such as ultraviolet light, has a high frequency and a great deal of energy. Amplitude is the height of the wave and gives a measure of its intensity, or brightness. Waves of large amplitude are brighter than waves of small amplitude.

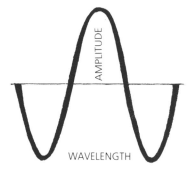

When a beam of white light is guided through each of four carefully placed prisms, (right), the colored beams that emerge contain the eighth color of the spectrum.

The number of colors in the spectrum is open to question: whether you see six, seven, or more depends on how exactly they are produced, how the overlapping colors appear, and what interpretation suits current theory!

Eight colors – including turquoise and magenta – are perceived by color practitioners (see p. 40). Magenta can be seen very clearly when looking through a prism on to white paper printed with black lines or bars. The magenta comes out of this juxtaposition of black and white, which mixes red with violet light.

The electromagnetic spectrum

The universe is bathed in energy. During the births, lives, and deaths of stars, galaxies, and other astronomical bodies immense amounts of energy are produced. Cosmic rays, gamma radiation, X-rays, ultraviolet rays, visible light, infrared rays, microwaves, and radio waves – collectively called electromagnetic energy – fill the inner and outer reaches of the known universe. Whether they appear to behave as waves or particles (see p. 33) the various forms of electromagnetic energy have two features in common: they travel at the speed of light and are made up of an electrical component and a magnetic component, which vibrate at right angles to each other.

For most purposes the energy can be considered as travelling in waves. The distance between successive waves is called the wavelength and the number of times a wave oscillates in one second is called the frequency. The rule of thumb is simple: the longer the wavelength of the energy, the lower the frequency.

The electromagnetic spectrum

The electromagnetic spectrum (below), embraces energies from cosmic rays to radio waves. They are graded according to wavelength, measured in nanometres. One nanometre equals one millionth of a millimetre. The spectrum of visible light falls between 380nm at the red end and 760nm at the violet end.

VISIBLE LIGHT

Cosmic rays Gamma rays X-rays Ultraviolet light Infrared light Microwaves Radar FM radio Television Short wave radio AM radio

10^{-7} 10^{-6} 10^{-5} 10^{-4} 10^{-3} 10^{-2} 10^{-1} 1 10 10^{2} 10^{3} 10^{4} 10^{5} 10^{6} 10^{7} 10^{8} 10^{9} 10^{10} 10^{11} 10^{12}

Wavelength in nanometres

Daylight

Fluorescent lamp
The spectrum of the light emitted from a fluorescent tube (above) is not full – there are more blues, greens, and ultraviolets than reds.

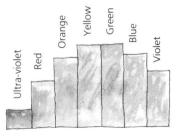

Full-spectrum lamp
The balance of the colors emitted by full-spectrum lamps (above) closely resembles daylight – reds, blues, and greens in roughly equal amounts.

All the forms of electromagnetic energy can be grouped into a spectrum (see p. 34). Cosmic rays have the shortest wavelength, the highest frequency, and the most energy. Consequently, they are the most damaging to living things. At the other end of the spectrum, radio waves have the longest wavelength, the lowest frequency, and the least energy.

Color and wavelength

The narrow band of energy that the human eye can detect fits roughly into the middle of the electromagnetic spectrum. The wavelengths of this visible energy extend from about 380 nanometres at the red end to about 760 nanometres at the violet end. Each minute shift in wavelength within this band of energy can be sensed by our eyes and interpreted as a specific color. In general, the colors are organized into the familiar visible spectrum – reds have the longest wavelengths, the lowest frequencies, and the least energy, while violets have the shortest wavelengths, the highest frequencies, and the most energy.

Beyond the red end of the visible spectrum there are the longer wavelengths of infrared radiation (which we feel as heat), microwaves (which we use in microwave ovens), and waves that we use for transmitting television and radio signals. Beyond the violet end there are the shorter wavelengths of ultraviolet radiation (which is essential for tanning the skin and for producing vitamin D in the body), X-rays, gamma rays, and cosmic rays.

Full-spectrum color

The energy of sunlight produces all the wavelengths of color, from ultraviolet through the visible spectrum to infrared, in a roughly even distribution. This is known as full-spectrum white light. We see the color of an object when our eyes interpret the wavelengths of the light it reflects. For example, a blue vase will absorb all the component colors of the white light shining on it except the blue, which it reflects.

When illuminated by sunlight the grass and leaves of a garden in spring display a range of greens, from the light, yellowish tones of the young shoots to the darker shades of the more mature plants. The fact that each different green hue shares the same power and vibrancy indicates the full-spectrum quality of sunlight, in which all the green wavelengths are present in roughly equal amounts.

People who spend a great deal of time in artificial lighting, which does not emit the same balance of colors as sunlight, are depriving themselves of nourishment (see p. 20). Although they can see sufficiently well they may soon start to suffer from a deficiency of natural light. This is borne out by people suffering from a condition known as SAD – Seasonal Affective Disorder – which is a depression usually brought on by the lack of sunlight during winter. An excess of inadequate artificial lighting can bring on similar symptoms. However, full-spectrum lighting, often incorporating ultraviolet light, prevents the development of SAD.

Color therapy lights are essentially full-spectrum lamps that are fitted behind colored filters. These filters are made from quartz, and are colored with gold, silver, or copper oxides to give a true, full-spectrum color. Gold produces reds, silver creates sapphire blues, and copper can color the quartz orange, yellow, blue, or turquoise. The filtered lights can thus produce colors of all the required wavelengths, frequencies, and energies. Ordinary artificial lights are unable to do this since they are more powerful in some wavelengths than in others. A cool white light, for instance, is weak in reds and violets, but strong in the colors between. When a red filter is placed in front of it, the resulting light is red but lacks the sufficient range of frequencies to be effective.

Extending the electromagnetic spectrum

Investigations into the mysteries of the universe have made scientists divide their subject matter into smaller and smaller parts. This goes against the elegant simplicity of the one world, one universe idea. However, recent advances in unified field theory have brought scientists back toward a more holistic approach to understanding phenomena.

Color practitioners have developed a different view of the electromagnetic spectrum, by linking light, sound, and matter (see right). These are all manifestations of energy, some of which have electric and magnetic fields around them, and others that do not.

From darkness to form
In the extended electromagnetic spectrum high-energy, fast-vibrating cosmic rays emerge from the darkness, followed by gamma rays, X-rays, and so on through the spectrum to the slow-vibrating radio waves. Beyond these, the energy loses its electromagnetic qualities and emanates as sound. Eventually, the energy vibrates at the level of molecules and atoms – the realm of matter and form. The emergence from darkness of light, sound, and form can be plotted on the extended spectrum. Their positions are given by the proportions of the "golden mean" (see p. 38).

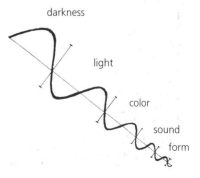

Just as music produces harmonic intervals, in which every note has a special relationship with each other, so all living things exhibit proportional relationships. Plants demonstrate these proportions clearly; look, for example, at the way a dandelion grows. Its leaves emerge from the centre with predictable spaces between them. The distances between these spaces are in the proportion of 1:1.6181, a proportion known as the "golden mean". In the early 13th century Fibonacci (c1170 – c1250), an Italian mathematician, recognized the "golden mean" relationship that was evident in plant, animal, and human structures and was the first to demonstrate this as a series of numbers, now known as the Fibonacci series (see Chapter Five). These patterns in nature are seen as evidence of the interrelationship of all forms of energy – whether visible or invisible.

Light and pigment

Color practitioners use both colored light and colored objects in their treatments, although colored light is more important because of its more powerful effect. Colored lights and colored pigments (in paints, dyes, etc) have different properties, based upon what happens when you mix

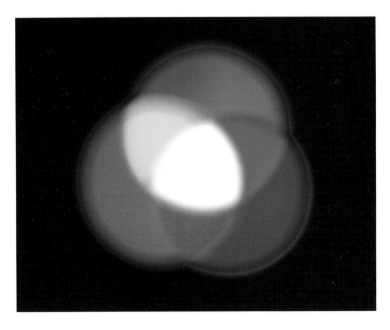

Red, green, and blue are the primary colors of light – if you mix them together in equal proportions you make white light. The colors of light are known as "additive", because they supply all the colors of the spectrum, which together make white. If you mix two primaries you make secondaries – red and green produces yellow, red and blue produces magenta, green and blue produces cyan (turquoise).

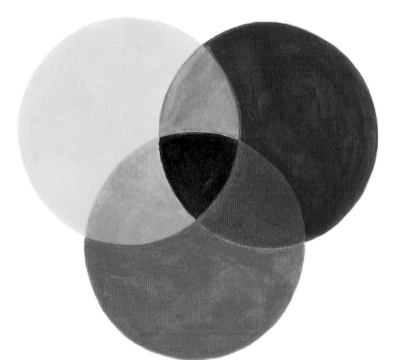

Mixing pigment colors

The primary colors of pigments, red, yellow, and blue, cannot be made by mixing any other colors. A mixture of these primaries looks black because together they absorb all the light that falls on them: a red pigment subtracts all the wavelengths from the light except red, which it reflects; a yellow pigment subtracts everything except yellow; a blue pigment subtracts everything except blue.

If you mix a pair of pigment primaries together you make the pigment secondaries – red and yellow make orange, red and blue make violet, yellow and blue make green.

Complementary colors

In the color wheel (right) the eight colors of the spectrum all occur opposite their complementary colors (see p. 40). For example, turquoise is the complementary of red, and yellow is the complementary of violet.

To maintain the balance in the body that is essential for health, colors are always used in their complementary pairs in treatments (see Chapter Six).

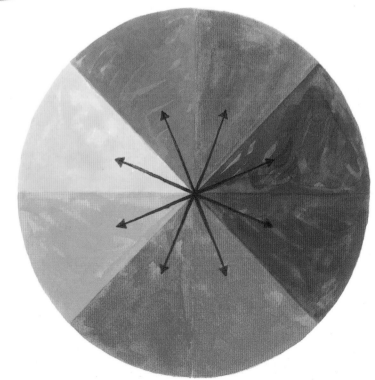

individual colored lights or pigments together. Primary colors are those that cannot be made by mixing any other colors. The primary colors of pigment are different from those of light (see pp. 38-9).

Wholeness and complementary opposites
In general, we try to categorize all objects and beings in the world and, in so doing, lose the sense of wholeness from which everything springs. Only by coming to grips with where we belong, instead of emphasizing how different we are, will we regain this sense of wholeness.

Everything belongs with its opposite – the north and south poles of a magnet, male and female, light and dark, yin and yang. The two opposites, like two halves, complement each other and create a wholeness *(see right)*. Moreover, each half contains within it the potential for the other half. Thus, the male contains the female aspect; the darkness holds the potential of light within; the yang yearns for the yin.

A color has its opposite, or complementary, too. Red and blue-green, yellow and violet, blue and orange are complementary pairs. But it is important to remember that every different hue has its complementary. The phenomenon of after-images illustrates complementary colors: if you stare at a red patch for about 30 seconds and then transfer your gaze to a white wall you will see a blue-green patch, the red's complementary. What is more, the quality of this after-image is a useful starting point for seeing colors in and around the body (see Chapter Four).

The importance of complementarity
One complementary color enhances the color of its opposite and when juxtaposed the pair makes the strongest contrast possible. Mixed together as light the two colors of a complementary pair balance each other and produce white. Thus, blue and orange light combine to make white light.

In the eight-color spectrum of color therapy, the complementary pairs are red and turquoise, orange and blue, yellow and violet, green and magenta *(see p. 39)*. Red, orange, and yellow are warm, magnetic colors, while turquoise, blue, and violet are cool, electric colors. Magenta and green are neutral in this respect. Complementarity is an

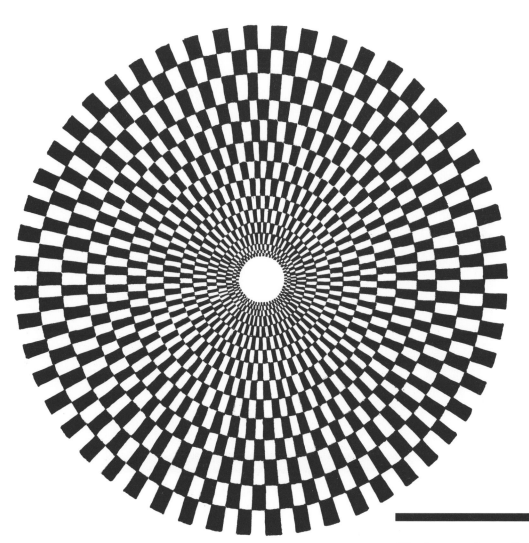

essential aspect of color therapy. A healthy body contains complementary colors in equal proportions, so balanced colors denote a state of good health (see Chapter Four). If you treat an ailment with one color without also using the balancing effect of its complementary you run the risk of making the ailment worse (see Chapter Six).

The interaction of opposites

In daylight, focus on the white circle in the centre of the diagram above. As you stare at it, you will see the inter-action between the blue and white areas as they appear to move and become overlaid with the colors of the rainbow. The two opposites create the whole spectrum.

For a stronger effect, a photocopy of this page will give you the true opposites of black and white.

feeling the effects of color

Human beings share their ability to respond to color with the world around them (see p. 20). This similarity connects us to the rocks, minerals, vitamins, molecules, atoms – to all solids, liquids, and gases. All matter, both organic and inorganic, is sensitive to electromagnetic radiation at all frequencies, and thus all things respond to the electromagnetism of light, and to its constituent colors.

This chapter explores the ways in which we respond to color – through the heart (intuition, emotion), the mind (brain, intellect), the body and its senses – and how we can enhance our color sensitivity. It follows the path of all our experiences *(see below)*, which are met first by the emotional response generated by the heart – the seat of intuition (see

Feeling, thinking, and action

The diagram (right) *illustrates part of the infinite cycle of intuitive and intellectual responses that lead to physical action. Following the path from the left, the heart gives the first, emotional reaction, which is followed by the response of the intellect, represented here by a crown. The crown is a symbol of perfection and its use in this context reminds us that our thoughts are perfect, although they may not be translated into perfect actions.*

The intellect controls the response of the body, represented here by a square, the symbol of manifested energy.

Throughout the cycle the balance is maintained between the response of the heart, mind, and body.

pp. 100–1). Once we have made an emotional, intuitive response to a situation or encounter our intellect is activated by the brain. Our immediate response is analysed by the intellect, which controls the subsequent response of the whole body. In the philosophy of Rudolf Steiner, this pattern of responses is summarized as "feeling, thinking, willing".

By learning to listen to your intuitive response you will enhance your sensitivity to color and maximize your color experience. In other words, you will develop your potential for working with color. You can strengthen your color awareness through techniques such as visualization, breathing, and movement, and enhance your ability to bring individual colors into consciousness.

The intuitive knowledge of color

Our first experience of color takes place in the womb. Early in childhood, color associations contribute to our consciousness. As we grow older we attach feelings, memories, and meanings to our experiences of colors, resulting in color becoming a feature of our sub-conscious. The association of particular colors with a happy, sad, frightening, or some other experience builds up our color preferences.

It is not too far-fetched to accept that our feelings about color become so closely attached to the memories – events, people, places – that they form a framework that we use to look at the world. Our recollections and feelings are "colored". They reflect our relationship with the outside world. Such is the basis of the psychology of color. In the same way that each color has physical and physiological implications for us all so, too, are there powerful psycho-logical, emotional, and spiritual connotations.

Our thoughts also color our minds at an even deeper level. Our responses to color are governed by deep-seated associations, which have been either conditioned by our experiences or inherited from our past. The phrase "I feel blue" indicates a cultural association between sadness and the color blue; "seeing red" refers to the color's deep-seated connection with anger. Expressions such as these indicate that we make intuitive connections between our feelings and the colors we use to describe them. Whether learned or inherited, the responses to colors are surprisingly similar the world over. This suggests the presence of universal color associations that are part of our natural connection with our planet.

It is sometimes difficult to accept these intuitive thoughts; and because the practical aspects of life drown our ability to be quiet and thoughtful, they prevent our intuition from developing fully. In many ways, experience and learning override our intuition. If you want to deepen your consciousness of color, the best way to begin is by relaxed contemplation, in which you are strongly aware of your feelings and in which you can trust your thoughts and find them valuable and worthwhile (see pp. 49-57). You can learn to heighten your intuitive response to encounters and experiences by allowing yourself the freedom to react to your initial feelings without analysing and substituting them with an intellectual response.

How shape enhances the power of color

Color practitioners work with colors that are presented in a particular form, or shape, because shape enhances the meaning of color. The logical, left side of your brain focuses on the form, whereas the more creative, intuitive, right side responds to the emotional impact of color itself.

By combining color with particular shapes, you allow the right and left sides of your brain to work together, thus enabling your conscious and unconscious mind to respond as one. Each color suggests its own shape – a shape that supports and maximizes the color's own energy, and provides it with a natural container. The shape of each color corresponds to the type of energy at work in the corresponding chakra *(see pp. 64-5)*. It also has internal energetic connections with the Platonic solids (see Chapter Five).

Color and the senses

Each of your five senses transmits information about the outside world to your brain, which processes it for meaning and relays it to your conscious feelings. Each sense can enhance your color experience but, equally, color enhances the experience of the senses. Traditionally, each of the five senses is linked with a color in a symbolic connection that has spiritual connotations.

Color and form

Look at the colors on page 47, and focus on your feelings about each color in the left-hand column. Then look at the right-hand column, where the colors are represented within a shape. Has the shape enhanced your feelings about the color?

Color without form

This is the color of the purest spiritual energy, that lets go all concerns and worries. The color of release, it transcends maleness and femaleness.

The color enhances self-respect and dignity. It gives a feeling for the intangible. Has female energy.

Blue has the energy of peace, relaxation, and openness. Its energy is female.

The color of freshness and cleanliness. Cool and springlike, it resembles the color of the leaves of spring flowers. Its energy is female.

Gives the experience of being free. Green is the color of balance; it stands mid-spectrum. Male and female qualities are balanced.

Yellow removes security. It enhances the need for the anchor because it tends to "lift away". Yellow increases the critical, judgemental faculty. Its energy is male.

Balance of red and yellow. Color of joy, movement, and dance. Its energy is male.

Stands for alertness, energy; it brings you into an awareness of the present moment. It carries the energy of "contraction", a male energy.

Color within a form

Signifies the aspiration to completeness. It is the symbol of perfection in sacred geometry.

Protects the blossom that is not yet fully opened, but that strives toward fulfilment.

Blue in the "opened" square offers itself up into relaxation. The shape is like a chalice. It is ready to move energy.

Focusing its energy downward, the triangle wants to integrate with the upward-pointing triangle, yellow, into the green circle.

The circle enhances the feeling of balance. The tension is equally shared throughout the shape — neither contracting nor expanding.

The energy of this upward-facing shape increases the insecurity of the color, which detaches from solidity.

The shape creates a dancing experience. It has a tendency to "lift off" — your own visualization keeps it in balance.

Creates strictness, security; a logical situation, a task to be done. The 90-degree angle is the angle of logic.

Sense	Color	Zodiac Sign	Gem	Element
Sight	Red	Aries	Onyx	Fire
Hearing	Yellow	Gemini	Gold topaz	Air
Smell	Green	Aquarius	Ruby	Water
Taste	Blue	Pisces	Sapphire	Earth
Touch	Violet	Libra	Aquamarine	Ether

Sight

Of all the senses, sight enhances your color awareness most. Its predominant effect takes place at the physical level, which is associated with the color red. Red helps you "pull yourself together" by enhancing your awareness of the "here and now". Generally, red has a contracting effect: "seeing red" refers to the very contracted or tense state of anger.

Hearing

By closing your eyes you remove the powerful sense of sight and enhance your powers of hearing. This helps to increase your awareness of color images produced by the sounds of music and speech. Equally, your most intense color sensations can make their presence felt as sounds. Sound can "shed light" on an experience, and allows the intellect to let go of ideas generated through sight. Hearing is associated with the element of air and the color yellow. This color symbolism illustrates the beginnings of traditional color connections between ourselves, the elements, and the energies of the planet.

Smell

Scents and smells indicate that a change is taking place. They are generated either when energies interact or when a chemical change occurs. The sense of smell is associated with the color green, the point of balance as the change takes place. The fact that the olfactory region of the brain is one of the first parts of the brain to evolve explains, at least in part, why smells can trigger strong memories and evoke early experiences of color associations.

Using sound to enhance light

The link between color and sound was familiar to the Druids who, at the winter solstice, retreated to their caves for three days. On the third day, each cave would be flooded with light and sound that seemed to have no source. By chanting, the Druids produced the full spectrum of harmonic overtones, which created a state of awareness that "let in" the full spectrum of light.

Taste

The experience of tasting delicious food or the full flavours of a drink is expansive – it takes you over and makes you vulnerable to the sensations. The expansiveness is associated with the color blue, the color that makes you relax. Blue acts as a taste enhancer when used to solarize water (see p. 116) – water in a blue glass (or a glass with a blue filter around it), left in sunlight for as little as 30 to 45 minutes will taste sweeter than before!

Touch

Your hands can heal by conveying more than the sense of touch – touching with care gives dignity, an invisible energy associated with spirituality. Because of this link with a higher level of consciousness, the sense of touch is associated with the color violet. Visually impaired people can interpret colors through feeling the density and temperature of the air that surrounds objects. By this "touch at a distance" people with poor sight can live in a world of color.

If you visualize violet when giving someone a massage, for example, you will help that person feel uplifted. By making color part of the whole experience you will improve the quality of your touch.

Enhancing your responses to color

Equipped with an awareness of your heart, mind, and body responses to color, and the knowledge that all your senses contribute to your color perception, you are ready to embark upon the practical techniques for enhancing your color feelings. The visualization, breathing, and movement exercises that follow on pages 50 to 57 will prepare you for working with the healing power of color, as well as guide you into the specific healing uses of the techniques that are described in the chart on page 101.

As a preliminary step in this process you should intensify your exposure to color and heighten your responses to it. To begin, try the exercise described on the following page. Talk about a particular color with a group of friends or fellow students. By identifying and strengthening your color associations you will become more aware of the characteristics of individual colors and begin to notice how they change the way you feel.

Talking about colors

Red and blue are the best colors to discuss first because their effects are so different and our experiences of them are often clear and plentiful. Sit in a circle and begin by describing the color red. You do not need to see the color, just keep it in your mind and let it "sink into you" as you speak. Then focus on your wider associations with the color, recounting your experiences and feelings briefly. Listen to the rest of the group expressing their feelings about the color and take in their thoughts.

After a few minutes you will notice that speech speeds up and the group members become more tense, as if anxious and on edge. Their breathing becomes more shallow and people generally feel ill at ease.

Talking about blue produces the opposite effect, almost one of lethargy. The members of the group speak more slowly and their breathing becomes deeper and slower. Examples of individual associations with the color take longer to emerge. Time seems to pass more slowly and eventually the group runs out of energy for the discussion.

Color visualization

The technique of color visualization enables you to continue the enhancement of your color sensitivity. You can then combine it with color breathing exercises (see p. 54) and finally with movements that help you to express the feelings associated with the different colors (see pp. 56-7). The end result will give you an intimacy with color that will not only prepare you for seeing a person's aura (see Chapter Four) but will also enable you to feel and work with the energy of individual colors for specific healing purposes (see Chapter Six).

In general, using your mind's eye for visualization helps you to balance negative thoughts – those that have lingered in your mind for many years tend to increase the ageing process because of the chronic tensions they produce. As a rule, use visualizations to accentuate positive feelings – use images of what you want to happen, rather than what you fear might happen.

The color red, in all its shades, from deepest crimson to palest pink, represents strength and vitality, and is energizing and stimulating. A red rose (right) is the symbol of emotional and physical love.

Visualization might be difficult to start with because it makes you feel awkward and the images are cluttered up with everyday thoughts. Use the simple relaxation (see p. 53) as a preparation for your color visualization. This enhances your concentration and enables you to focus more clearly on the images. Being relaxed also has the advantage of allowing your body to absorb color readily, and this contributes toward the healing process.

Simple relaxation

Lie on your back on the floor. Make sure that your body is straight and your chin tucked in. Your legs should be slightly apart and your hands by your sides, palms facing upward.

Relax your mind, and let any thoughts float up into the atmosphere like beautiful balloons, and then gently disperse. Then bring your concentration into your body. Starting with your head, use your mind to work down your body to your feet.

Gently let go of any tension and feel yourself starting to relax.

Then, on the next inhalation, bring your arms up over your head and stretch your whole body.

Exhaling, bring your arms down to your sides. Repeat this twice. Now gently roll on to your side and sit up.

Preparing for the exercise

After the relaxation, sit comfortably, and follow the simple visualization exercise given below. You can work with any colors for this exercise (see p. 54). The example below describes a visualization using blue, and its complementary, orange.

Simple visualization

Exhale slowly and close your eyes. Inhale gently, and imagine that you are sitting by a blue lake. The sky is blue above you. As you exhale, think of looking at the intense orange of a large marigold flower. Feel the calmness of the blue fill your body.

Repeat the exercise a few times, then sit quietly for a few moments before you get up. The breathing technique is described in more detail on page 54.

Visualization-meditation

To take color visualization a stage further you can meditate upon an inner story. An example of such a story is told on page 53. Familiarize yourself with it or ask a friend to read it to you. Alternatively, imagine a story of your own.

Think of this visualization as a way of travelling "out of your body". Before starting, you must feel assured that you can return safely. To do this, relax (see above) and sit upright, then look at the space around you. Remember the colors and shapes that you see. Feel protected by the space, and ready to return there after your visualization.

Exhale slowly, close your eyes, and follow the story below in your mind's eye.

At the end of the story, take a deep breath and bring your thoughts back into your body. Return to the vision of yourself as you were before closing your eyes.

Finally, imagine a ring of light that contains a cross of light. Think of your eight chakras (see p. 65) and, starting from the top – the crown chakra – visualize the ring and cross of light working as a golden key to "close" each chakra in turn. This protects you from the shock of re-entering your normal consciousness.

The inner story

I walk into a market place on a sunny afternoon. It seems strangely empty and no one seems to see me.

I am drawn to the church at the end of the square. The door leads down into a deep crypt where the red eternal flame burns in front of an altar. I let this red flame take me inside its strength, even power, and remain there experiencing this feeling of life-giving energy. The image of God the Father comes to mind.

After a while I stand up and walk up a few steps to a hall where the light is orange. Many people are dancing, moving. There is joy and laughter. I am only an onlooker and no one acknowledges my presence.

A flight of stairs leads me up into the main aisle of the church. The vaults reflect a yellow light; all seems so detached; it feels lonely, almost empty; I can't stay there long and I look for an exit.

Behind the altar a door leads into a grassy field. The green restores my balance and I walk on the grass toward a forest.

The color under the leaves of the trees is turquoise: fresh, pure, and making me immune from any kind of influence. It feels as if everything is just beginning.

I walk through this forest and stand before a blue lake. Some blue hills across the water give me peace. I am relaxed and very calm.

As I look across the lake, a beautiful being bathed in a violet light moves toward me. I am overcome with a dignity I have not experienced before. In its hands burns a beautiful magenta flame. This flame is free and lets go of all density or substance.

The figure does not change in size as it comes toward me. The violet and magenta increase in strength and uplift me, filling me with respect, not just for this being but also for myself. Now it stands before me and speaks in a clear and beautiful language: "You are to take this light and carry it in your heart; it is the light of pure love. Let go of all past burdens."

As I accept this light, naturally and without hesitation, it is still in the hands of this being whom I recognize as my higher self – pure, free of burden, and just complete love. There are no strings attached to this love – only love. "Take this light into your everyday life and give it to all you meet." The being (and it feels as if it is myself giving myself the permission to go back into the world) retreats across the lake and I am nevertheless aware that it is also with me at my own calling. The words "World without end," sound within me.

The flame in my hands penetrates the blue of the lake and shares this cool, relaxing peace. I walk back through the forest – the trees and shrubs smile as I give them my flame of love, the flame of magenta. It is a very pure, very light magenta, almost white. I am not alone any more. The grasses, the little flowers, the rabbits come to me as I cross the green field.

I did not notice all this before. I return to the church; the yellow arches are still detached but they shine now as if they were golden and absorb my flame of light. I descend into the orange hall and offer my flame of pure magenta to the people who come to me. Each one now has one flame also. I say to them: "Share it always, share it or else it will go out." To be joyful and dancing with the light of love seems so natural.

And now I descend into the crypt, where I can accept the red of the life energy, which resides in the base of our being, through which we can create the future children to maintain the Earth and its life. I suddenly realize that my magenta flame of love is not only in my hands but penetrates all the cells of my body; nothing is untouched by this flame of love.

Humble yet proud, I ascend the stairs and enter the market place, which is busy with many stalls. I go to each stall holder and give them my light of love. I had not noticed until now that the light in my hands is only the centre of a vast radiance all around me and that as I give it away it radiates even stronger each time I share it.

Now slowly return to your normal waking state, (see left) using a deep breath, and closing your chakras.

The calmness that comes from meditation on the blue of water beneath a blue sky (right) can be experienced through the simple visualization on page 52.

Color breathing

Breathing does more than bring oxygen into your body and remove the carbon dioxide from your blood; it sustains and revitalizes your spiritual energy. Your breathing provides a continual interaction with the world around you. Concentrating on your breath also allows you to clear your mind of unwanted thoughts. Furthermore, rhythmic and stable breathing provides you with a firm platform from which to explore your conscious and subconscious self. Breathe fully, and rhythmically, from deep inside your abdomen.

Solar Plexus

Simple breathing technique
Lie down, or sit up with your spine relaxed and straight. Breathe at a rate that is comfortable for you. Do not try to elongate the inward and outward breath and do not hold your breath. Just establish a natural rhythm, focusing on the breath until your mind is calm, and free of unwanted thoughts.

In your mind's eye hold a positive image of yourself; for example, picture yourself at a time when you felt particularly well or happy. Now bring a color to mind.

You can either go through the whole spectrum of colors, or choose a particular one for its healing qualities (see right).

When you have decided on your color, breathe in, visualizing the color entering your solar plexus and spreading throughout your body just beneath the skin. If you wish, imagine the color penetrating a specific part of your body. As you breathe out, visualize the complementary color. Use the information that follows to guide your color choices.

Red *Breathe in red for vitality. It brings energy and increases sexuality, strength, and will power. Breathe out turquoise.*

Orange *Breathe in orange for joy, happiness, and fun. Breathe out blue.*

Yellow *Breathe in yellow to increase your objectivity and intellectual powers. Breathe out violet.*

Green *Breathe in green to cleanse, to feel more balanced, and to combat tumours. Breathe out magenta.*

Turquoise *Breathe in turquoise to counteract inflammations and fever, to strengthen the immune system. Breathe out red.*

Blue *Breathe in blue for relaxation and peace, and in cases of sleeplessness. Breathe out orange.*

Violet *Breathe in violet to increase self respect, and for feelings of dignity and beauty. Breathe out yellow.*

Magenta *Breathe in magenta to let go of any obsessional images, thoughts, and reminiscences. Breathe out green.*

Movement

The beautiful gestures of eurhythmy introduced by Rudolf Steiner at the beginning of the 20th century provide a series of simple movements that help your color visualization. Eurhythmy was developed as a performance art, but has a therapeutic use, and can be practised in order to enhance the feelings associated with each color.

The movements developed from the contrasting feelings associated with "light" and "dark". Yellow is the lightest color in the spectrum, and the color most like the sun. The position that represents this light is very open, with the arms reaching up, as if toward the sun. Conversely, the darkest color, indigo, is characterized by the arms held low, and the body folded downward. Between these extremes the characteristics of each color style the position. Eurhythmy always involves movement that follows the shapes already made by the body, so none of the color positions is static. You pursue the color's form by following it through; and moving the arms.

Moving from light to dark

Begin by lifting your arms up and slightly to the sides. Relax your chest and keep it "open", as if to receive the light (see position 1, right). Then bend one knee, lifting your heel to help the movement. Let your knee curl in toward the other leg. As you do this, fold your body forward, relax your arms and lower them as much as you can, gently closing them across your body, as if shutting out the light. This position represents dark blue, the color of darkness (see position 2, far right).

Position 1   Position 2

Red

Red is much darker than yellow, but contains more activity. From position 1, dip your hands down in front of you, then push them up briskly but smoothly in front of your face. The color red is a very dynamic color and the movement is correspondingly fast and firm. Its movement is "penetrating", sometimes almost aggressive. It helps you "cut through" any problems.

Green

Green is the color between yellow and blue in the spectrum of colors. The movement explores the middle region, with the hands held out to the side. Maintain the height of your arms as you move them around, and step both in straight lines and circular shapes, reflecting the balance between "open" and "closed" movements.

Yellow

Yellow is the brightest color of the spectrum, but not as brilliant as white light. So, from position 1, lower one arm very slightly forward, and think of it as a shaft of light. Lower your other arm down behind you, completing the diagonal with the arm that faces up. Move gracefully forward and back in straight lines, following the diagonal direction of your arms.

For colors that are made from a combination of two others – orange, for example, contains red and yellow, and violet is made of red and blue – the position of the arm and the movement of the body should reflect the characteristics of both. As you move, the extreme positions of each color "give up" something of themselves, to produce a flowing movement of a single color.

CHAPTER FOUR

color energies in the body

This chapter focuses attention on the subtle color energies that surround your body all the time but usually go unnoticed. More than that, it looks at how energy emanates from your body itself. And it shows how you can begin to learn to perceive this energy as a color signal, which is a direct indication of the health of both body and mind.

A cautionary note is called for here. From the information in this chapter you can learn only how to start to increase your color perception. In order to see color images with absolute clarity, you have to use techniques that involve going into deep meditational states that alter your brainwave patterns. For this you need the instruction and direct supervision of a qualified practitioner. You can, however, practise the techniques of dowsing described here (see p. 70), in order to detect the color energies of the spine. This will give you an introduction to experiencing color energy and prepare you for further guidance.

Energy input and output

The energy we need for life comes not only from our food and drink but also from the electromagnetic radiations of the sun, and the invisible forces of galactic space. The effect of the moon, alone, is greater than you might think. Its gravitational influence over the tides is well documented; less well known is the fact that some surgeons are cautious about performing surgery around the time of the full moon, because of the moon's tidal impact on the flow of blood in the body.

We do not find it difficult to think of plants drawing on sunlight in the process of photosynthesis, using the energy from the rays that penetrate their leaves to combine the carbon dioxide from the air with the water and trace elements drawn up from the earth, and so to produce the material for growth and reproduction. In this process, the sunlight energy is necessary to the plant for the synthesis of food.

We human beings are also bathed in light from the sun, which affects our bodies directly. The light penetrates our skin and muscles, even our skull (see p. 20), to bring warmth and produce chemical changes in body tissues. It also triggers hormonal effects that alter the pattern of our growth and reproductive processes. Thus there is an essential interaction between ourselves and the energy that surrounds us.

Haloes and wings

Familiar "halo" shapes traditionally surround the heads of Jesus and the saints in paintings during the time of Fra Angelico and Botticelli in the 15th century, and other Italian artists dating back to the 12th and 13th centuries and before. These, and the wings of angels, are an historic acknowledgement of the perception of more than just the physical human form.

The halo and wings are not, however, the prerogative of saints and angels. They are potentially present in the auras of all humans.

Everything on earth takes energy in, and releases energy. The process of life and growth involves this exchange of energy with the environment – an input and an output. Part of the output is a unique energy field that exists around every living being, including human beings. Think of a human being as having not only the immediately visible physical body, but emanations of this subtle "output energy" that surround the body, but are not visible (or only visible to some). They form a protective zone of transition between your physical body and the outside world. This area is called an aura. It holds your life energy, reflects your state of health, and filters out and takes in the energies of the universe. The aura is continually moving and pulsing, and this free movement of energy is what keeps you healthy (see also Chapter Five).

Minerals, plants, animals, and humans all have their own auras, which differ in their complexity and color ranges (see *Evolution of the aura, below*). Minerals have a white aura around them, plants a golden one, while the aura surrounding animals is indigo blue. That of humans is multi-layered, and multi-colored. This complexity represents the added dimension of consciousness, together with all aspects of our physical, mental, emotional, and spiritual functioning; it is expressed in eight (or possibly more) subtle layers (see pp. 62-3). The vibrations and colors of the layers of a human aura alter as a result of internal changes in health and consciousness and the effects of external energies (see pp. 76-7), although the overall shape of the aura remains more or less constant. These are natural phenomena, indicating the normal changes that take place in healthy, living things.

Evolution of the aura

Before the existence of matter, there was darkness. Then a slowing, or contraction of cosmic energies yielded light energy. As it slowed, it produced color, then contracted into sound, and finally into matter (see p. 37). Where the energies contracted very quickly, they formed dense, solid matter, such as minerals and crystals; those energies that "drew in" more slowly gave rise to living matter – cells, plants, animals, and finally produced favourable conditions for the emergence of human life.

All matter releases energy. Matter that was formed by a quick contraction of energy releases its condensed energy very slowly. Dense, solid objects have still auras, which are difficult to perceive. Human auras are mobile and fluctuating.

The human aura

The aura extends all around every human being (facing page). Always in a state of flux, its size, shape, and color depend on the precise condition of the individual. To those people who are gifted and those with special training, the aura is easily perceived, and so can be used in color therapy, providing a useful diagnostic device and a guide to treatment.

Quality of colors in the aura

The colors of the aura are clear and luminous; they are indescribably fine emanations of energy.

You can see for yourself what this special quality of light is like by looking at a solid printed color for about 15 seconds, in order to saturate your vision. Then cover the color with an opaque sheet of white paper. The new color that you see now – which is the complementary color to the original – has a luminescent quality. This is similar to the quality of color that is visible in the aura.

Structure of the aura

Immediately surrounding our physical self is an etheric sheath, extending three to four inches (8-10 cm) around the body and following its form. It is the spiritual blueprint from which the physical body develops. Under normal conditions its color is a very pale magenta (it is absolutely white when the person is spiritually highly evolved). Those who communicate in a peaceful and relaxed manner produce a bluish energy that colors the sheath. Good teachers are surrounded by a cobalt blue etheric sheath. A violet note suggests someone with dignity, who may, therefore, be involved in religious work.

Around the etheric sheath is the aura itself, a three-dimensional ovoid extending several feet in all directions, in volume about 22 times larger than the human form. The aura contains layers of color just like the rainbow and these layers are continuously moving, interpenetrating each other with their clear, pure color. These movements respond to environmental inputs as well as shifts in thought, feeling, and physical wellbeing. The layers of the aura are a pre-manifestation of the whole person. Each corresponds to a different aspect of the human function.

The human aura

The first layer, next to the etheric sheath, is **red.** Red is the densest color and relates to the physical body and sexuality. The **orange** layer, next to it, is the energy of the life force, the metabolic body. These two layers are very closely linked. The metabolic body maintains the physical body during sleep and provides the energies of breathing, heartbeat, and blood circulation. It also nourishes the involuntary nervous system. It is sometimes referred to as the etheric body. The **yellow** layer, also known as the astral body, corresponds to the solar plexus and the emotional energies: the soul of the individual. Next to yellow is the **green** layer, representing the ego, personality, and the capacity to think and make connections between the physical individual and the subtle, finer, spiritual energies of the aura. Green is the color of balance; this is the area of exchange between the ego and the higher self. The **turquoise** layer that follows the green links up with the higher mental, or super-mental, inspirational self. The **blue** layer is the model for the causal body, or motivation; it holds

Sharing an aura

The shape and size of your aura depends on your feelings and your state of health. When you meet a real friend, you feel warm and "expansive" – and your aura grows accordingly. The opposite happens when you meet someone you dislike; your aura contracts and "withdraws". If you are both in the expansive state, you each move into the other's aura, absorbing its energies and, to some extent, leaving the imprint of your own aura there.

in it the plan for life that we would ideally love to live. Beyond this is the **violet** layer – the higher self, the bodyless body, the true essence, and the greater consciousness. The last layer that is discernible is the **magenta,** representing the spirit self, the identity, the eternal being.

Chakras

The auric layers are "breathing" energies around the human being that correspond to living energy. By contrast, there is another energy comparable to rays of light, shining both into and out of centres in the body. These centres are known as the "chakras". Sanskrit teachings from Tibet well over 2000 years ago talked of three chakras. Later, the Tibetans recognized five, and since then seven and more have been acknowledged. Eight chakras, corresponding to the eight colors of the aura, are described below.

The chakras are lens-like structures that collect and strengthen the light that surrounds us. Each chakra has a greater and lesser centre (see p. 65). Whereas the layers of the aura that surround the human body produce a "container" energy, the chakras provide the "content" of the container. These two energies are complementary, and work together both to create and to maintain life. The container energy of the aura is the feminine aspect and the ray-like chakra energy provides the masculine aspect of these complementary energies.

The colors and functions of chakras

Magenta The crown chakra relates to the pineal gland. Magenta is the color of the eternal, spiritual self, made up of the energies of perfection. The centre of spirituality, this chakra connects you to an infinite intelligence.

Violet The brow chakra, also known as the third eye, transmits the energy of the pituitary gland. Known in yoga as the 1000-petalled lotus flower, it is the centre of creative visualization, and gathers instruction from your higher self.

Blue The third, throat chakra is centred at the energy of the thyroid gland. It is the centre for creative expression through sound, and as such is significant in matters of communication and truth.

Turquoise The chakra of the thymus gland is very closely linked with the heart, and connected with a generosity of life and love.

Green The heart chakra is the centre of love and harmony. This is the area for a person's soul to shine through. Green is the color of balance.

Yellow The solar plexus, like a sun, is the light that has descended into the nervous system. From here you are sensitive to situations. It is the centre of human recognition and self worth. Unresolved situations create stress here.

Orange The sacral chakra relates to the adrenal glands, and is strongly influenced by genetic patterning. Its connection is less spiritual, more earthly. Physical movement, wellbeing, and joy relate to this chakra.

Red The base chakra is connected to passion, life energy, sexuality, and the power to create.

Chakra	Sanskrit name
Crown (pineal)	Sahasrara
Brown (pituitary)	Ajna
Throat (thyroid)	Vishudda
Thymus ⎫ Heart ⎭	Anahata
Solar plexus	Manipura
Sacral (adrenals)	Swadisthana
Base	Muladhara

The chakras

The eight chakras, corresponding to the eight colored layers of the aura, lie in line with the spine, in the etheric sheath (see below).

Traditionally in Tibetan teaching the thymus and heart are one energy, so these two chakras share the common Sanskrit name.

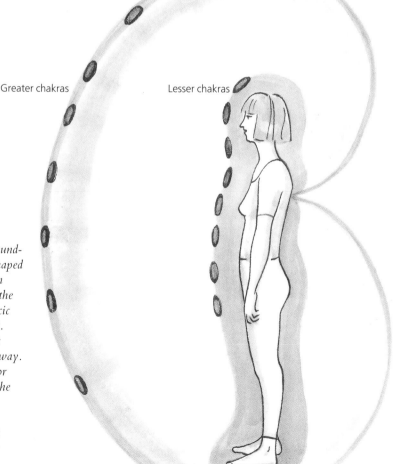

Greater chakras

Lesser chakras

Chakra energy

From the side, the energies surrounding the body produce a kidney-shaped profile. A funnel of energy, even finer and more transparent than the aura, penetrates to the 5th thoracic vertebra, at the level of the heart. This is where the energy of light guides each individual along the way.

The position of the smaller, or "lesser" chakras corresponds to the edge of the etheric sheath, about 3½ – 4ins (9-10cm) from the body. The greater chakras are at the edge of the aura, about 32ins (45cm) from the body.

Detecting color energies

Early attempts to measure and detect aura and chakra energies were made in the late 19th and the first half of the 20th centuries. This interest was a response to technical advances, including the early use of electrotherapy, and to claims by scientists and clairvoyants who reported seeing luminous emanations surrounding the body.

Walter John Kilner was a physician and surgeon at St Thomas' Hospital, London. After his appointment in 1869, he became director of the one of the first X-ray departments. His attempts to design an instrument that would allow him to see the luminous emanations of the body led to experiments with a dye known as dicyanin. By looking through a lens coated with the dye, he could perceive light in the ultraviolet range. The apparatus became known as the Kilner screen, and it made visible a blue-grey band of light that extended six to eight inches (15-20cm) around the body, with a second band of almost vaporous light extending outward. He found that fatigue, disease, or mood could alter the size and color of the radiation. Magnetism, electricity, and hypnosis also altered the image.

In the 1930s and 1940s, a Russian technician, Semyon Kirlian, observed tiny flashes of light on the skin of patients receiving electrotherapy. He devised equipment to reproduce this effect and recorded the result on photographic paper. One of his most significant findings was that every person produces a unique energy pattern.

Human potential

These attempts to measure invisible human energy patterns, to a large extent the product of their age, made important advances in the acceptability of the idea of the human aura. But no instrument has been able to detect more of the aura than the etheric energy that immediately surrounds the body. Human beings, however, have the potential ability to perceive the multi-colored human aura directly. The pituitary gland is thought to be the organ responsible for this perception. A few people retain the gift from birth, but most lose it. Color practitioners receive training in how to become aware of auras and to dowse for color in the body. They may use any of the techniques described on the pages that follow.

Energy in the aura and the chakras
The human aura is three-dimensional, surrounding the body in all directions (see p. 62). Similarly the energies surrounding the body that funnel into the chakras come from all directions (see p. 65).

In this two-dimensional representation, the aura is shown flat on the page, while the chakra energies are focused in from above the page. Where the chakra energy shines directly into the aura the colors of the chakra energies and the layers of the aura mingle, creating pure and luminous colors.

Accepting color energies
Start by thinking about the colors, and accept the possibility that you, too, can perceive them. Imagine perceiving the colors of the aura. Allow the subtle energies into your consciousness. If you can do this without feeling that you are "pretending" to experience the colors, you will probably start to become aware of color sensation. Not necessarily immediately; it will be easier for some than for others. But once you have really accepted the possibility, you become more receptive to the color energies. Go back to the exercise on page 40; and remember that the quality of the colors is transparent and luminous. Practise the exercise until you have seen the whole range of complementary colors with the same luminous quality as an aura. After that, it is a matter of letting these colors in; allow yourself to see them, and these subtle energetic vibrations can become clear to you.

Perceiving auras
Learning to become aware of auras involves voluntary and controlled changes in brain states. You can start to learn the techniques for perceiving auras yourself (see pp. 68-70), though a good teacher will always be your best guide. The techniques are simple, and closely connected with the relaxation exercise described on page 53. But you will need guidance in returning from such altered brain states. They should not be attempted on your own.

Altered brain states
You, as a human being, are able to change your brain state at will. The following description gives you an idea of the different levels of brainwave patterns that you can achieve, and which you need to experience in order to become conscious

of the colors of the aura. Four levels of brain activity are described here, all of which can be recorded on an electro-encephalograph. The brainwaves become longer as the brain pulse decreases. These changing levels of consciousness can be accessed through meditation, which makes an excellent and safe introduction to altering the pulse rate of the brain.

Slowing the brainwaves

In an anxious state, mental activity can reach 34 cycles per second – the *higher beta* rate. The brain pulse rate during normal human activity is 21 cycles per second, the speed of the normal *beta* rhythm. The level below *beta* is the calm *alpha* state, at 13 cycles per second. This alpha state is the natural level of brain pulse rate for animals.

Below *alpha* is the *seta* state, when your brain is slowed to about 8 cycles per second, and you are even more focused and calm. At this point solid objects start to look transparent. If you slow your brain one stage further, to 5 cycles per second, you are in the *delta* state. You can no longer differentiate between hearing, seeing, and feeling. Time and space become interchangeable. You can at once feel an experience and "see" it as if you were on the outside. Perception no longer depends on the "sight". In this state you need help to be drawn back into more normal states of consciousness.

Consciousness and your aura

The change in your consciousness is also reflected in your own aura. The normal, *beta* pulse rate produces the typical multi-colored aura. As your rate slows to *alpha*, the aura shows a blue overlay. At *seta*, the blue gives way to gold, and if the *delta* state is reached, the aura is almost white, lightly tinged with magenta. In effect, you are moving through all the levels of consciousness of the evolutionary process (see p. 61).

The aim is to slow the brain pulses. This has the effect of finely tuning your perception to the higher vibration level of color energies. As your brain pulse slows, you become more receptive than in your normal brain state.

As a result of moving into a meditative state some people suddenly find themselves able to "see" what they previously could not. This can also happen as the result of a shock – whether good or bad – which detaches your personality and soul from your physical self. In this detached state, you are open to "seeing" things that you would not normally see. By being more "opened up" to the energy of light, you allow its colors to influence you.

Asking permission

Looking into someone's aura is a very personal matter. Always ask permission before entering into this world of subtle messages. You may well experience a distorted image if you go into it without permission.

Color in the spine

The aura and the chakra system are two ways of expressing the presence of color energies in and around the body. A third way of looking at these energies is as they might appear in the spine. It is possible to look at the spine of the human structure as carrying within it a memory of its own stages of evolution.

This process is recorded as deep-seated memory within the spine and the nervous system. The vertebrae, which house the central cord of this system, and the skull, can be divided into five sections, each representing one of these evolutionary stages; the physical manifestation, the metabolic processes, the emotions, the intellect, and the spirituality. Each section contains eight vertebrae, each with the concentrated color energies of the eight colors of the spectrum (see p. 71).

Sensing colors in the spine

If you have not yet experienced the ability to "see" the colors that surround people, you can tune your senses to the vibrations of color through dowsing. The most well known style of dowsing is with a water diviner, a forked stick that helps to concentrate the energies below ground level. The pendulum is almost as familiar for this (see below). But one technique that is relatively easy to learn and very simple to use, is to use your finger to sense the amount and type of activity in the body, through the vertebrae (see p. 70). Everyone can learn to dowse and this makes the diagnosis of color energies in the spine a relatively simple activity. And once you begin to work in this way, you may find that it makes you more sensitive to working with color in other ways, too.

Working with a pendulum

Choose a pendulum that feels comfortable to hold. Find out first which way it moves in answer to your questions. It can answer "yes", "no", or "do not know". The movement may be circular, from side to side, or forward and back. To find out, sit down, holding the pendulum so it hangs about

Using the pendulum

Once you have established how your pendulum moves for "yes", "no", and "do not know", you can use it for dowsing.

Hold the thread between your fingers, focusing your mind on your questions. Remember that these must be clear, and require only a "yes" or "no" response.

Pendulum materials

A pendulum can be made of metal, wood, or a crystal, held by a thread or a very fine chain 9-12ins (23-30cm) long. The finer the thread, the less it will resist movement.

two inches (5cm) above your knees. Keep your hand with the pendulum very still. Then ask, "What is my yes?" Allow time for the pendulum to start its movement, and then remember the result. Before the pendulum stops moving, ask "what is my no?" Let the pendulum give its own direction. Do this several times daily, until you are confident about what every movement means.

Working with a pendulum is a very personal thing; always dedicate yourself to the work, and do it for the benefit of your friend or client, with no other thought or purpose. Keep your pendulum for your own use only.

Dowsing with your finger

The spine chart (see facing page) allows you to record the active energies in the human spine. All you need is a "witness", such as a lock of hair, a photograph, or a signature from your friend or client. The witness should be written on the back of the spine chart, or simply placed behind, in the case of a photograph or hair, and the chart laid on the table. It is wise to remove any written documents or printed material from any drawer underneath.

Dowsing the spine

Use the middle finger of your left hand (your right hand if you are left-handed) and start at the top of the chart (right). Let your finger hover about half an inch (1cm) above the paper. Work down the chart, vertebra by vertebra, and allow yourself to feel the sensations. You will feel nothing over the inactive vertebrae. The active ones will give you a hot, cold, repelling, or tingling sensation.

Record the result as you move down the chart, noting the strength of the response – strong, medium, or weak.

Spiritual area
The eight fused bones of the skull receive messages from our higher, spiritual self. They are not used in diagnosis because of the difficulty of interpretation.

Mental area
Color in this area of the spine relates to the ego, thoughts, memory, and intellect.

Emotional area
These vertebrae carry information about the astral realm, or soul, your relationships, feelings such as joy, love, hate, and anger, any emotional turmoil, heartbreak, and the way we react to the world around us.

Metabolic area
These vertebrae represent issues that are connected with your physical-etheric life force, your household, routine tasks, rhythmic metabolic processes, including the digestive system, food, toxins, and drug and alcohol consumption.

Physical area
This area can provide information about your physical being, sexuality, obsessions and habits, physical ailments, survival and reproduction, exercise and sport, and other regular activities.

7 cervical vertebrae

12 thoracic vertebrae

5 lumbar vertebrae

Sacrum

Spinal diagnosis
The system of analysing color in the spine gives yet more opportunity to diagnose the condition of the body and mind (see pp. 72-3), and another way of allowing color into the body, for healing purposes.

Order of colors
The order of the colors within each section is the same, following the colors of the rainbow, from magenta at the top, through to red at the bottom of each section.

Color intensity
The intensity of the colors increases toward the bottom of the spine, because this represents the physical functions, where the colors are more contracted, and therefore more dense.

The colors of health

In a balanced, healthy human being, the colors in the spine turn up repeatedly, in groups of eight, from top to bottom (see p. 71). In a healthy spine, the color in a vertebra has a counterpart, which is its complementary color. The original color and its complementary are connected at an energetic level. Where the color energies in the spine exist in complementary pairs, their energies are balanced (see p. 90). These vertebrae may also be described as "matched", or "bridged". Where the complementary color does not appear, the original color remains "unbridged", and represents imbalance in the body (see Chapter Five), rather like an energy still looking for somewhere else to go.

The chart below describes the significance of the colors in a healthy spine. The information makes specific reference to the four sections of the spine: the mental, emotional,

Colors in the healthy spine

MAGENTA

Mental	Emotional	Metabolic	Physical
"Let go" or "change" You are making efforts to change and let go of old memories.	You are letting go of old feelings, and allowing your feelings to change.	You are managing to leave behind domestic habits that no longer apply, and changing your eating habits where necessary.	You are making efforts to change your activities that no longer apply, and to be free of the influence of others over your lifestyle.

VIOLET

Mental	Emotional	Metabolic	Physical
"Dignity" You are paying due respect to your personal mental activities.	You accept and respect your own feelings as being good and dignified.	Your home feels like a dignified place. You are treating everything at home, including food, with respect.	You respect your body and behave in a dignified way.

BLUE

Mental	Emotional	Metabolic	Physical
"Relaxation" Your mind is relaxed and peaceful.	You feel peaceful and relaxed.	Your home life is relaxed; meals are eaten in peace.	You undertake your activities and physical work in a relaxed state.

TURQUOISE

Mental	Emotional	Metabolic	Physical
"Immunity" You are independent and immune from other people's thoughts.	You are coping well; other people's feelings do not impinge on you.	Your immune system works well; you make sufficient energy available to it.	You are behaving freely, not following the will or obligation of others.

metabolic, and physical. The color depends on the level of activity in each vertebra (see p. 70). In reality, it would be very unlikely that all colors would show up as being active at one time. This is because daily rhythms continually alter the activities within the body (see p. 77). And as it is normal for human beings always to be in a state of progress toward a new equilibrium, some parts of the spine are likely to be more active than others at any one time. By making a series of charts, each on different days at different times, a practitioner can build up a full picture of the spinal energies and their patterns.

In practice, dowsing usually shows up activity in about half the vertebrae of the spinal column. The activity of each color is summarized below by a word or expression that describes its characteristics.

GREEN

Mental
"Balance" You have a balanced mind, and you are not letting your work affect your home life, or vice versa.

Emotional
You have a balanced relationship with your partner, and you are at ease with the social structures of your life.

Metabolic
Your home life is stable, and you are balancing periods of activity and relaxation.

Physical
Your actions are balanced. You act at the right time.

YELLOW

Mental
"Detachment" You can think clearly and make sound judgements.

Emotional
You are able to detach yourself from your own and other people's feelings to see them objectively.

Metabolic
You can look at your home objectively, and appreciate or criticise the way you have created it.

Physical
You are able to act according to the needs of the moment.

ORANGE

Mental
"Joy" Joy and happiness fill your thoughts.

Emotional
Your heart is open and joyful, giving you enjoyable emotional exchanges.

Metabolic
Joy and pleasure at home help the digestion and give strength to the whole body.

Physical
You are able to enjoy all the physical activity that is needed of you.

RED

Mental
"Strength" You have the energy to think, and to carry out all your mental requirements.

Emotional
You have enough strength to be open emotionally.

Metabolic
Your energy for your home life means that it is in good order; so, too, is your digestive system.

Physical
You are coping well with your daily physical activities.

The body in balance

The five functions of the human body – spiritual, mental, emotional, metabolic, and physical – are always exchanging energies with each other. This never-ending movement is the best indicator of life, and while energy is being exchanged and maintained in balance, the body remains healthy. The smooth and continuous flow of energy in your body depends on your ability to acknowledge each of the five functions. This creates a unity in your being that means you can draw on all your energies in order to achieve your aims – rather like a rowing team pulling together in unison.

The idea of acknowledging all the aspects of your body's functions sounds simple, although it is probably harder for most people to carry out than you might think. If, for example, you are particularly good at producing ideas, but not so good at seeing them through, you should learn to acknowledge your physical activities more – do some gardening, for example, and get your hands dirty! This helps to "ground" you, improves your connection with the physical aspects, and will connect your mental and physical processes, enabling you to carry out your ideas. The aim is always to create a flow of energy through the emotional, mental and physical aspects of yourself. An imbalance in the flow will create problems at all levels. For example, fear can create anxious thoughts, which can lead to problems in the metabolism. You can only achieve a balanced flow by maintaining a healthy level of activity in all aspects of yourself.

The Spinal Diagnosis Chart (p. 71) is a particularly good indicator of these connections. The energetic swirl of color in the human aura also mirrors the quality of the energy flow through the body. The colors of the aura in a healthy person have a characteristic glow and brightness (see p. 67). For example, the red energy of the base chakra (see p. 64) is bright and clear in those people whose physical and sexual lives are healthy and joyful.

Red can very easily lose its beauty in this respect when the mental and emotional energies are focused only on physical gratification. The red is then not fully imbued with the transmuted energies from the other energy centres of the body and becomes very murky. In cases of rape, the red,

Working in the garden, you will absorb the healing color energies of nature, which vary with the changing seasons (right). An hour a day spent in a natural environment is a wonderful tonic.

sexual energy of the offender's aura is tainted with black. All centres, when not operating at their peak, including those occasions when human intentions are not "pure", become darker and unclean looking.

The active vertebrae of the spinal column are constantly maintaining an exchange of energy, and while this exchange works to produce an equilibrium, the body is in a state of health. Naturally, it is impossible to hope for a perfect state of health, because of all the external and internal changes that are going on all the time. The body is always working toward that state of perfection, rather than achieving it.

Variations in the aura

The continual flux in the energies of the aura is accentuated by normal daily activities (see right) and sleep patterns, as well as the ageing process. When you are asleep, your "container" energy (the rings of the aura) is very strong, and the activity of the chakras is less pronounced, making the ray-like energy that shines into and out of the chakras very fine in appearance. In the awake state the opposite is true. Your "content" chakra energy becomes stronger, while the surrounding layers appear finer by comparison.

During childhood and until puberty, the reds and oranges are dominant in the aura, and the time is correspondingly active and playful. By about 12 years, yellow starts to dominate, then from 24-36 years and 36-48 greens and turquoise appear more, highlighting balance and clear health, which serve family life well. The blues, violets, and magentas are more evident after 48 years of age. Blue and violet are the colors associated with teaching and serving, when we can share some of the knowledge and skills gained through life. Magenta, the dominant color from 72 years onward, is the time for letting go – time for the next generation to take over.

Temperament and the aura

In addition to the daily changes in the natural ebb and flow of energies, and the those changes created by the ageing process, differences in temperament produce corresponding highlights in the color energies. Rudolf Steiner distinguished the same four types of temperament that Hippocrates (c460-c377BC) first described. Sanguine types, connected

Designs for movement and health

The above pattern is reproduced from a ceiling in Cleveland Hospital, England, where terminally ill cancer patients are treated. It combines the healing colors of blue and gold with a pattern that creates both movement and direction.

The pattern entices the viewer to follow its form, a representation of the head (at the top) and the rest of the body (below), with the heart in the middle. The effect of this is to encourage movement throughout the body – the antithesis of illness, decay, and stagnation. This movement enlivens the whole person and helps to reconnect the mind, the body, and the emotions.

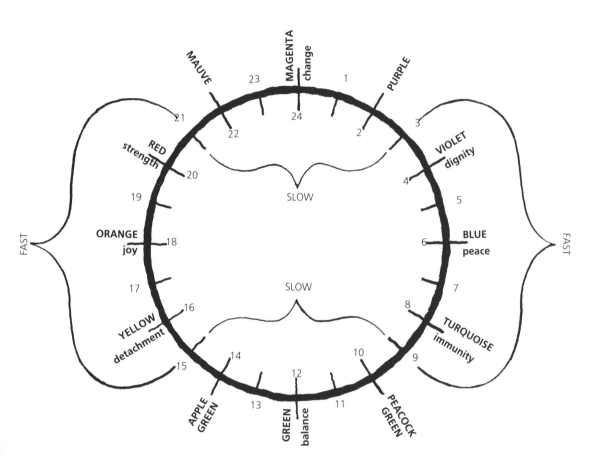

The diagram shows a circular clock-face with 24 hour markings and associated colors:

- MAGENTA change (24)
- PURPLE (1, 2)
- VIOLET dignity (3, 4)
- BLUE peace (5, 6, 7)
- TURQUOISE immunity (8, 9)
- PEACOCK GREEN (10, 11)
- GREEN balance (12)
- APPLE GREEN (13, 14, 15)
- YELLOW detachment (16, 17)
- ORANGE joy (18)
- RED strength (19, 20, 21)
- MAUVE (22, 23)

SLOW (top and bottom), FAST (left and right)

with the element air, make light of problems. They are good planners for long-term work and their aura is yellow-dominant. The melancholic pays attention to detail and is good at putting plans into practice. Prone to sadness, and sometimes "unable to see the light", the melancholic's color is blue, connected with the element of water.

The choleric type, associated with the element of fire, sometimes acts impatiently, and often before thinking. Red is the dominant color. Patience characterizes the phlegmatic – connected with the earth element and the color green. The phlegmatic person waits for things to happen, on the basis that "the mountain will come to Mohammed".

Daily rhythms in the body

The rhythms of the day and night affect the energy flow in your body, producing changing levels of activity. The daily cycle of 24 hours is divided into intervals of two hours. Each of these highlights a style of activity that is associated with a particular organ, and corresponds to a color. A further pattern is superimposed on this two-hourly rhythm: the hours between 9pm and 3am represent a general slowing of energy. Between 3am and 9am energy levels increase, then ebb again until 3pm. After this, the activity of early evening begins.

CHAPTER FIVE

feeling off color

As you progress through life, you will inevitably experience phases of good health and bad health. Your physical, mental, emotional, and spiritual development is the product of your genetic patterning and your life experience, including the food you eat and the quality of the environmental input. Even your thoughts affect the way you feel. This delicate balance of possibilities means that sometimes you may undermine your health very easily; at other times you will be well equipped to deal with life's changes.

Color therapy tests and diagnostic techniques are all based on the belief that illness is predictable from personality analysis. The thought processes are the origin of all disease, which may then become manifest in the emotions and the physical body (see facing page). Mental and emotional developments cause changes in your color energies, so these are reliable indicators of illness that could become evident at a later date. Specific changes in the aura, or in the color energies of the spine, relate to specific problems that may exist. Because of this, color treatment can detect and work on these problems before the illness manifests in the body. This approach differs from Western medicine, which can only begin to treat symptoms that have already penetrated into the physical body.

Illness and its diagnosis

This chapter looks first at the significance of illness and then at its diagnosis through color. It puts illness into a context; the product both of physical changes sometimes connected with bacteria, viruses, and other agents of disease, and of mental and emotional imbalances that arise throughout the normal course of life.

Color therapy uses a variety of techniques for diagnosis, some of which you can learn with little training. All of them are described in this chapter, and some can be mastered from the information given; others need additional training. Color practitioners may be trained in some or all of them. Some practitioners work on aura perception, using changes in the shape and color of an aura to give information on a condition (see pp. 86-9). Others dowse to detect the quality of color energies in the spine, then analyse the balance of these energies by means of a chart, where all the information

Transforming your negative thoughts

If you are entertaining negative thoughts, or clinging on to negative attitudes, confront them, and you will be in a better position to let them go. If these thoughts go unrecognized, they tend to turn up in the emotional area as bad feelings, and much more deeply anchored than before.
Relax, let go of all your tensions throughout your body. Breathe normally, then surround yourself in the color magenta, which allows you to let go of your thoughts. By letting go of this negativity, you emerge strengthened, and ready for the next step in your personal development.

The development of illness

Your journey through life can be illustrated as a spiral. Where there has been a change in your mental state (point A, left), when you again find yourself in a similar situation (on the next turn of the spiral, point B) you will encounter that change at an emotional level. If your emotional response is resolved, you shift into a new pattern of life and continue on a slightly altered spiral path (point C). If your emotions are left unresolved you will meet them again in the future, but this time at a metabolic level (point D). Once the problem manifests in your metabolic processes, your life force is weakened; the road back to health will be a longer one.

is recorded (see pp. 90-2). Psychological tests (pp. 94-7) can supply additional information on your personality and needs. In using these tests, you have strong indicators of your health tendencies.

The Color Reflection Reading (pp. 94-5) monitors the way your personality and life events are affecting your health, and directs you in the use of therapeutic color techniques. The Lüscher color test (p. 96) also produces a detailed personality analysis. Art therapy (pp. 96-7) looks at the interaction between personality and health by analysing paintings. Each section includes a discussion of the individual use and value of these diagnostic tools.

Health and movement in the body

Your body is in a continual state of flux. Changes occur at every level within you and your health is intimately connected with your ability to accept these changes. Movement of every kind is natural in a healthy being. Without movement, development would not take place.

If the movement in your body – from the beat of your heart, to cellular activity – becomes sluggish, your body will cease to function efficiently and you may become ill. If this happens, accept the illness as a challenge, as an opportunity to "move on", both mentally and physically. By doing this, you progress toward a more healthy body and a more highly developed mind. Illness is a learning process, a lesson on the way to greater consciousness.

The ideal state

Your body and mind have a "memory" of the ideal state, deep seated in your subconscious, but also available to your superconscious, or higher conscious self. By getting in touch with these parts of your mind, for example by the methods of relaxed visualization described on page 52, you can begin to find the pattern of your personal needs. By looking into yourself, you can begin the process of healing.

The challenge of illness

Pain, or a diagnosed disease, is bound to make you start thinking about how you can regain your health. Doctors can provide doses of sophisticated drugs, all of which affect your physiology, sometimes altering your moods as well. They may make the symptoms go away, but frequently bring with them their own side effects and only provide a temporary respite from the disease symptoms. Real cures demand the patient to take part in the healing process, otherwise the treatment is merely a "cover up" for a cure.

By looking into yourself to understand your illnesss, you may isolate habits connected with your diet, your sleep, or your physical environment, that prevent you from functioning at your best. You may, equally, examine your thoughts and feelings – for these are at the root of all chemical changes in your body. Negative attitudes such as guilt, hatred, revenge, not being able to forgive, and holding grudges, affect not only mental activity but are soon reflected in your emotions and your physical body. Just by taking these first steps, you will put yourself in a closer relationship with your body and mind, and you may be able to address thoughts and behaviours that were upsetting the healthy flow of your body's energy.

Understanding yourself

The path to health is different for everybody. People with apparently the same illness may nonetheless experience different symptoms, while people with the same symptoms may need to follow a different path to health.

Energy in, energy out

Your ability to keep energy moving within you depends not only on the free passage of energy in your body that unites your mental, emotional, and physical aspects, but also on taking energy in and letting it go. Think of your body as continually breathing – not only the breath that fills your lungs, but a pulsing energy always flowing in and flowing out. Your health and personal development depend just as much on this continual exchange of energy in and out of your body, as on the free circulation of energy inside you. Ultimately, the result of all movement ceasing is death – no movement into or out of the body.

Children's development
Children up to the age of puberty are accumulating energy from the instream. After puberty, they have a strong enough sense of self to give, in the sense of being generous with their own spirit. Expecting predictable standards of behaviour from children before this age, for example by trying to "show off" a child's particular ability on request, damages a child's need to reveal him or herself at the appropriate time. This behaviour also exhausts children's energies, thus robbing them of the strength they need to build up inside.

Cosmic etheric energy

The energy that you take in originates from cosmic energy. This is the life force that underlies your ability to breathe, eat, grow, have feelings, and think.

The physical energy from food and drink is just part of the energy that sustains us in life. Both cosmic and physical energies are types of etheric, or "life-supporting" energies. While food provides the physical, or metabolic etheric energy, life itself depends on cosmic etheric energy.

Instream

The intake of cosmic etheric energy depends partly on your genetic tendencies: you are born with a capacity to welcome the outside world or to turn your back on it. Your experiences as a child and adolescent also have a strong influence on this instream of energy. If you as an individual have been fully accepted for what you are, then you will be open to the cosmic, life-giving energies that surround you. Cosmic energy streams in to happy people more than it does to those who are sad. In denying themselves their own happiness, sad people also deny themselves the strength and vitality that could support and replenish them.

Outstream

The outstream of energy depends on how well your own expressions of energy are met by others. If others try to curb these energies in you, then you may suffer from depression and frustration. The free flow of your energy includes the ability to express yourself freely, and not to be constantly undermined.

Working with a counsellor

Whatever type of color therapy you go for, the first stage is to talk to the practitioner in order to build up a picture of your personality and needs. The particular questions depend on the individual situation – the reasons for you starting treatment in the first place, and the skills and experience that the practitioner brings to the therapy session.

The two main questions that the practitioner will ask in your introductory counselling session are, firstly, how your behaviour (or your condition, if you have a specific ailment) and feelings change throughout the day. When are you particularly active? When do you feel particularly tired or sluggish? This question helps give the practitioner some insight into the color energies that are working well – where the colors in your aura would be pure and bright – and those that might need attention during the therapy sessions.

The second question is about your favourite and most disliked colors. Following this, the counsellor tries to find the origins of these likes and dislikes, by asking questions about situations that might have given rise to the good and bad associations. The reason for trying to identify these good and bad psychological associations is that both can create an imbalance in your day to day color exposure. You may well avoid a much needed color, just because of an unpleasant past association. The aim is to regain an equal acceptance of all colors.

A third question might arise, about your favourite pastimes. The answer to this tells the counsellor how wide the gap is between how you spend your time and how you would like to spend it.

The counsellor may go on to discuss various aspects of your life, corresponding to the four sections of the spine (see p. 71). These questions are not always easy to answer; they need thought and insight into aspects of your life that you may not have previously considered. The key question is "How well do you acknowledge the mental, emotional, metabolic, and physical areas of your life?" Your answers not only help the practitioner to interpret your spine chart (see p. 91). They will also enable you to see for yourself whether you accept or reject your life at any of those levels.

For example, in the metabolic region of your spine, the relevant issues surround your home life, the regularity with which you conduct your domestic arrangements, and the amount of care you put into them (see p. 71). If you acknowledge the importance of these issues, it will mean that the energy in that area of your spine should be pure and bright, and the colors that appear in that area are likely to be balanced, or "bridged" (see p. 72). If you do not acknowledge the need to give the metabolic area of your life this sort of attention, then you are likely to be blocking the energies in that area, and this may create discolorations. The blocked energies prevent the smooth and free flow of energy throughout your whole body; your mental, emotional, metabolic, and physical areas are no longer well connected and the balance goes out of your life. Eventually, illness may result. By diagnosing this sort of problem before the onset of any illness, you can receive appropriate advice concerning your domestic life, and put right the problem before it even becomes apparent. Your answers also tell the practitioner how ready you are to make changes in your life.

Underlying all this is the need for you as patient to want to co-operate with your counsellor. Counselling can help to elicit information that you may want to share, but that you find difficult to articulate. But no professional counsellor will make you give information before you feel ready.

Case study

David suffered from severe migraine, and the color blue came up repeatedly from the Spinal Diagnosis. Light treatment with the color blue was unsuccessful, and he resisted using blue visualizations. For some reason he was unable to respond to the color.

By the fourth treatment, the only solution seemed to be to talk to David about his past, and to see if blue had an emotional attachment that was blocking the treatment. David told me that he never wore blue clothes, nor decorated his home with blue; he was uncomfortable with the color. I asked him if he had been frightened or upset at any time when the color blue was present. He recalled a train crash in which he was involved when he was eight years old. The train was de-railed. It was night time and he fell out of his bunk. Above the door of the compartment was a small, blue nightlight.

Having recognized the root of David's problem with the color blue, I encouraged him to try to overcome it, and suggested that, by accepting the color again, he might well find relief from his migraines. It represented an energy in him that he was not acknowledging. After practising by relaxing into the color blue, subsequent treatments were more successful. David was able to accept its healing powers. A few months later, he chose to redecorate his office in shades of blue. He reported that his migraines had all but ceased.

Diet and your aura

Even the food you eat has an impact on the quality of colors in your aura. Highly processed foods, and especially those that are packaged, sealed, and stored, lack energy and produce a correspondingly thin aura. If you eat too much meat, your aura becomes denser. If you have a very faint aura a practitioner may advise you to eat more fish or meat.

A child has a naturally shiny, luminous aura (right), with red as the strongest color, reflecting the natural activity and playfulness of childhood (see p. 76).

Changes in the aura

Your aura fluctuates, as already said, as a response to changes both within you and in the environment. The two main fluctuations are in the color and the shape. Most of the color changes result from changes within, and signal a slowing, a speeding, or a blocking of energy in the body. The changes in shape are usually inflicted from outside. The size of the aura may also change in both cases, contracting or expanding, depending on how free you feel to behave naturally, or whether you are being constrained. Many of the small changes rectify themselves through your own natural adjustments. More severe changes can be dealt with by using color breathing and visualization; treatment with colored light may be needed for more problematic alterations in the aura.

Color changes

The rainbow colors of your aura breathe, expanding and contracting, so that all the colors start to dance. In health, the colors are pure, bright, and quite dense, or strong. Happiness creates sparkling movement, and a slightly shiny effect. Feelings of love overlay the aura with the colors of amethyst and rose quartz. Sadness represents a low energy state, and the colors become slightly dimmer, even dull. Dreamy people also have faint auras; they are less grounded physically, so the colors are correspondingly less solid.

The two most common discolorations of the aura are brown and grey. They are the results of "energy in" not equalling "energy out" (see p. 82). A grey discoloration suggests you are creating a barrier to an energy input of some description. This could be at the mental, emotional, metabolic, or physical level. At the mental level, it might be an unwillingness to take on somebody's ideas; at the emotional level, fear of an emotional involvement; at the metabolic level, a lack of desire for food.

The position of the discoloration in the aura corresponds to the level of the problem. Problems at the mental level are seen in the outer layers; emotional, metabolic, and physical problems come progressively closer to the body. The discoloration also relates to the position of the fine, ray-like energy of the chakras (see pp. 64–5). For example, fear of an

Using discolorations
for diagnosis

*The chart below lists the significance
of energy blockages in the aura.
These are represented by brown
discolorations (holding on to energy)
and discolorations of grey (blocking
energy input).*

emotional involvement will show as grey in the green layer
(which is connected to the heart) and also grey in the area of
the heart chakra.

Brown signifies "holding on" to energy that needs to be
let go. Even having a cold discolors the aura in this way,
and represents a negative attitude, such as "Even if this is
bad, I shall hold on to it". Someone who freely takes, but
rarely gives, is more likely to have this brown discoloration
of congested energies.

Chakra/Spinal area	BROWN (holding on to energies)	GREY (blocking energy input)	Treatment Color
CROWN/MENTAL	Obsessional thinking		MAGENTA YELLOW
		Thoughtlessness	
PITUITARY/MENTAL	Obsessional images		DEEP BLUE ORANGE
		Lack of images	
THROAT/MENTAL	Too talkative		VIOLET YELLOW
		Silence/autism/ perfectionism	
THYMUS/EMOTIONAL	Mean		ORANGE BLUE
		Overgenerous/not able to receive	
HEART/EMOTIONAL	Closed/unresponsive		TURQUOISE RED
		Too open/indiscriminate	
SOLAR PLEXUS/EMOTIONAL	Fear		BLUE GREEN
		Overconfidence	
SACRAL/METABOLIC	Weak sex drive		RED BLUE
		Strong sex drive	
BASE/PHYSICAL	Lethargy		RED GREEN
		Overactivity	

Shape changes

The most likely cause of shape changes to the aura is shock.
A shock may make your aura shift away from your head; it
may also move away from your heart, leaving both head
and heart unprotected. The effect of this is to separate your
spirit self from your physical sensations. If the shock is severe

enough to shift your aura away from your heart region, your emotions will no longer feel connected with your body. You might feel as though you are about to faint, or even as though you are on the verge of a nervous breakdown.

A shock that is not quite so severe, such as witnessing a bad car accident, may regularize after about 24 hours. During that time you feel vulnerable, insecure, and unable to accept any form of responsibility. You lack connection between your personality and your own mental activities.

A mild shock, such as cutting yourself, or falling down a few steps, may shift your aura briefly away from your head. Taking a deep breath is usually enough to bring your protective aura back into place. You should also try visualizing the color blue, and using your color breathing techniques (see p. 54), breathing blue in, and orange out. End with a green visualization to regain a feeling of balance.

Electro-convulsive therapy can also move the aura away from the body. The etheric sheath maintains the life systems of the body. Color treatment can help re-unite the chakra energies and their bodily counterparts, and reconnect the soul and spirit to the physical and life forces.

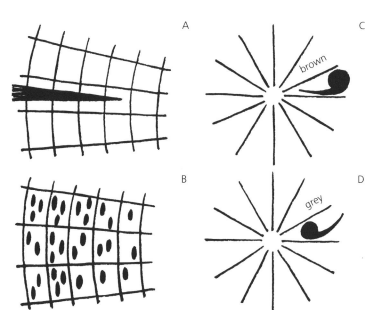

Unhealthy patterns in the aura
The use of hard drugs can create wedge-shaped areas in the aura that have no color, and therefore appear black (see diagram A and p. 90). This indicates a serious depletion of the body's energy.

Flecks or shadows in the aura (diagram B) are usually a reaction to more minor toxins, such as alcohol or nicotine. If no more toxins are ingested these flecks will disperse within about 4 hours. However, if the intake increases the shadows in the aura will increase.

Brown discoloration of the aura (diagram C) results from an inability to let go of energies (see facing page). Conversely, a grey area (diagam D) indicates a barrier to accepting energies (see p. 86).

Negative emotions can also alter the shape of your aura, although not on the scale of the shock reaction. Hate and jealousy produce a jagged edge to the auric layers, which weakens the structure and effectively means that your protection is undermined.

Hard drugs also give the aura a similar jagged edge, which becomes irreparable if bad drug habits continue. Like a log of wood that dries out, the aura can begin to "split", making wedge-like areas of depletion. These are colorless intrusions into the aura that can, over a period of time, reach the centre, leading to complete exhaustion. The wedges affect the chakra energy, and may deplete any of the glands. The colors in the aura that surround the body become cloudy.

Sensations

As you dowse, you may feel sensations of heat, cold, tingling, or repulsion. Tingling is a good sign of vibrant health, while heat, cold, or repulsion suggest that your energy is out of balance. An experienced practitioner takes this into account when making a spine chart.

Color changes in the spine

Dowsing the spine can give you a very clear indication of the color energies in the body. By dowsing with the middle finger, as explained in Chapter Four, and feeling the reactions, you can then record the information on a spinal diagnosis chart (see opposite page) in order to create a clear picture of health.

As you work down the vertebrae on the spine chart on page 70, your finger registers responses of different strengths, indicating which of the vertebrae are currently active. Record the strength of the sensation on your spinal diagnosis chart (see below and opposite page).

Key to response strength

very weak	−	−
weak		−
weak to medium	−	0
medium		0
medium to strong	0	+
strong		+
very strong	+	+

Typically, about 16 out of the 32 spinal vertebrae are active, sometimes as many as 18, rarely fewer than 11. If your dowsing finds more than 18 active vertebrae, it may be that you need more practice to distinguish sensation from non-sensation. However, some people who are exhausting themselves may show up more than 18 active vertebrae.

Spinal diagnosis chart

Working on the spine chart

Color the active vertebrae on the spine chart, using the colors indicated by the vertebrae. The rainbow pattern of eight colors is repeated in each section of the spine.

Mark on one side of the chart the strength of the response.

In order to locate the complementary colors with ease, it is useful to draw the complementary color of each active vertebra in a column by the side. Then, starting with the uppermost active (colored) vertebra, look for that same color in the column, starting at the bottom. Your aim is to join the complementary color as far down the spine as possible. Then take the next colored vertebra down and do the same thing. Repeat this, always choosing the complementary farthest away, until you have joined, or "bridged", all the complementary colors. You are then left with colors that are active, but unbridged. These indicate colors for treatment (see Chapter Six).

Refer back to the chart to see which of these colors gave the strongest signal. That is the color for treatment. Date the chart.

Strength of response

Mental

Physical

Emotional

Metabolic

Color of active vertebrae

M
V
B
T
G
Y
O
R
M
V
B
T
G
Y
O
R
M
V
B
T
G
Y
O
R
M
V
B
T
G
Y
O
R

Complementary color

Date/time

The chart produces a unique pattern for each individual. Because of the energy changes in the body during the day (see p. 77), you should record the time of the test. Make a new spinal diagnosis before any treatment, in order to record the changes over time.

Once you have filled in a spinal diagnosis chart and joined the pairs of complementary colors (see p. 91), you can begin to look at what the colors mean. You might have several pairs of bridged colors, and several unbridged colors. If all the colors are bridged, it suggests a healthy exchange of energy within the body. The links between the mental, emotional, metabolic, and physical aspects of the body represent an acknowledgement of those functions and a free flow of communication between them. A link between the mental and physical areas is particularly good because the connection from top to bottom works also through the emotional and metabolic layers. Unbridged colors suggest the treatment colors; use the one that gave the strongest signal (see Chapter Six).

Using the information from the spine chart, you can transfer the details on to a simple résumé, which will help you see how well the energetic connections are working. The résumé allows you to summarize several spine charts, and show you the changes over time, or the progress of every treatment session. You can also use your summary of a series of spine charts to show up the underlying personality characteristics.

Using the spinal diagnosis chart

Mark the bridged pairs as shown (right). This highlights how many sections are involved in the connection. Mark the unbridged colors in their color, or in a symbol or short form for the color (as right).

Unbridged colors indicate a lack of that color in that section of the body and need treatment. If there is more than one unbridged color, enhance the unbridged color that has the strongest signal (for example, mark it with a cross). This is the color to use in treatment.

The number of columns used for the summary of each spine chart will depend on how many vertebrae are active, and how many of these are bridged. Remember to mark the date and time of the spinal diagnosis.

Mark the bridged pairs and then the unbridged colors start with the uppermost active vertebra and its pair.

Summary chart of the spinal diagnosis

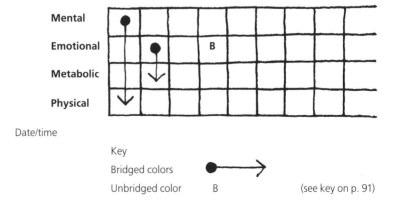

Date/time

Key

Bridged colors

Unbridged color   B   (see key on p. 91)

Analysis

The ideal connection is between complementary pairs in the mental and physical regions of the spine. Some color pairs may be bridged within a single section. This indicates a healthy acknowledgement of the activities of that section, but a less free flow of energies overall.

Once you have completed the summary chart, look back at the strength and type of signal you received from the unbridged colors while dowsing. If you have found more than one unbridged color, use as the treatment color the one that produced the strongest signal.

Refer back to the descriptions on page 71 to see how each section functions. With practice it becomes straightforward to analyse the connections between these different sections. The following case studies show how to build a picture from the spine chart.

The meanings of the unbridged colors

Mental	Emotional	Metabolic	Physical
Magenta You are not letting go or changing your old thoughts.	**Magenta** You are not letting go of old feelings.	**Magenta** You are ignoring your changing needs in food and household.	**Magenta** You need to change your daily or weekly plan of actions.
Violet You have no respect or dignity for your own mental work.	**Violet** You lack dignity, and are ashamed of your feelings.	**Violet** You are treating your home and belongings with disrespect.	**Violet** Your body feels undignified.
Blue Your mental process is not relaxed; you lack peace.	**Blue** You are not relaxing, and cannot enjoy your emotions.	**Blue** You take no time to eat, to study, or to enjoy your home.	**Blue** You are not giving yourself enough time to do things peacefully.
Turquoise You have no immunity from other people's thoughts.	**Turquoise** You are unable to be immune from the feelings of others.	**Turquoise** You have a digestive weakness, or inflammatory condition.	**Turquoise** You are too easily influenced by those around you.
Green Your mental process lacks balance.	**Green** Problems in personal relationships may be causing you upset.	**Green** Your home life lacks balance: the same might apply to your diet.	**Green** You are doing things without order or plan.
Yellow You lack objectivity because you do not detach yourself.	**Yellow** You cannot detach from other people's emotions.	**Yellow** Look after your calcium metabolism; you may have an arthritic condition.	**Yellow** You are doing things which are now no longer necessary.
Orange You experience no joy or happiness doing mental work.	**Orange** You lack joy and happiness.	**Orange** This may be an indicator of anorexia.	**Orange** You experience no happiness or joy in your activities.
Red You have no energy or strength, and are easily tired.	**Red** You have no strength or energy for expressing your feelings.	**Red** You lack energy because of bad digestion.	**Red** You lack sufficient physical strength or energy.

Personality assessment

Personality assessments help give you insight into your patterns of behaviour. This may, in turn, suggest how your health might be affected, and how you might benefit by working with color, once you have this knowledge.

Color Reflection Reading

This technique is a practical way of working with the psychology of color and produces straightforward color advice. It was devised in 1985 by Dorothy and Howard Sun and is presented in a shortened form here to show how the technique works. Refer to Living Color in the Resources section (p. 124) for more details. Color Reflection Readings take about one hour and require the interpretation of a color counsellor. Other color diagnoses and treatments use the range of techniques described in Chapters Five and Six.

Eight colors are presented in shapes (see p. 47) printed on white card, in two rows. By making three color choices, you can access your innermost thoughts and feelings directly. The Color Reflection Reading uses color as a new language to reflect information related to our physical, emotional, and mental wellbeing.

Analysis

The first color represents your true essence, your basic personality. The second color relates to your present condition at a physical, emotional, mental, and spiritual level. It reflects your deep, subconscious needs, and your main challenges. The third color indicates how you might take your next step, to a new level of personal awareness.

The exercise

Choose the three colors that you prefer at this moment. Do not think about it; let your intuitive mind do the work, and choose your colors straight away, rather than allowing your judgements to interfere. Forget about your "favourite" colors and any associations that sway your feelings. Place the three chosen colors separately in front of you in order of preference.

The significance of your color choices

First position
You are an initiator, a pioneer, a creator. Active and physical. You need to harmonize your emotions with your logic to obtain the equilibrium you seek.

Second position
Your challenge is to energize yourself, but without exhausting your resources. You need to reduce domination and work on expressing your warmth and friendship.

Third position
You want to feel active, but you are exhausted. Try to replenish yourself and quieten your system.

First position
Joyful and ebullient. Sometimes tired through over-activity. Listen to yourself, learn to be still, and trust your basic instinctive nature.

Second position
Your greatest challenge is to make time for yourself, and find stillness in body and mind.

Third position
You may have inwardly withdrawn. You can be more courageous and confident. Try to be willing to take more risks than usual.

First position
You tend to search constantly for information. Good with words, You can be dominating. Your work probably carries responsibility.

Second position
The challenge is to think about your physical self, not just your mental ability, so that you can express the energy relevant to now.

Third position
You need to work out how to expand your mind, perhaps through education, to bring optimism into your life. A holiday in the sun could help.

First position
A personality full of balance, sometimes lacking in spontaneity through over-caution. Neat and efficient, with an affinity for natural materials.

Second position
Your main challenge is to express your emotions, and to come to terms with emotional hurts. You may be acting out of unfulfilled need.

Third position
By making more contact with people, you will lift your spirits, and feel more valuable, less serious. Guilt and inertia will also diminish.

First position
You are imaginative and full of fresh ideas. You make yourself clear, you are popular, and can deal with demanding situations. You have insight and are spiritually orientated.

Second position
Learn to control the demands of others and give yourself time to reflect. You may need to cleanse your body, mind, and emotions to prevent toxification and illness.

Third position
You welcome the challenge of change as part of a personal transformation, although this can produce fear, turmoil, and upset.

First position
Gentle by nature, you are also reliable. You make people feel secure. You value truth and honesty; at times your inward searching is too self-absorbed, making you isolated.

Second position
Your strength is your silence and knowingness; your challenge is to express yourself more directly, in order to avoid inertia and melancholy.

Third position
Be flexible enough to take a more earthly, practical attitude toward daily life. Use relaxation to restore yourself, but not as a *modus operandi* or means of escape.

First position
A mixture of red and blue, you apply your spirituality in a grounded way. Aesthetic, artistic, and with a sense of ceremony, you do not always feel sure that you will achieve your vision.

Second position
Although you are likely to be in a position of authority, your challenge is to ask for acknowledgement. Otherwise you may become negative about responsibility. Persevere.

Third position
Violet encourages you to use your creativity, and to share it with others. Practise using your innate capacity for faith, intuition, and wisdom.

First position
Kind, co-operative, and friendly. Often very mature, with a deep understanding of life. Likely to be working in the caring professions.

Second position
Your challenge is to balance giving and receiving because you tend to neglect your own needs. Learn to receive as well. Nurture yourself; respect your own needs.

Third position
As you strive to blend the basic life forces (red) with heavenly power (violet), you risk developing a grandiose self-image. Let go, and allow the gentle part of your nature to shine.

Case study

Harry is 29 years old, of average build and about 5'10" (1.78m) tall. He is a computer operator; intelligent with a quiet disposition. He wore a faded **brown** shirt with **navy blue** trousers. When Harry made his color choices, **blue** was his first choice, **green** his second, and **orange** his third.

First position – BLUE

This color speaks of a quiet, gentle, and peaceful individual, someone whose tendency is to be self absorbed and introspective. "Blue people", like Harry, value qualities such as truth and honesty and believe in approaching life carefully and without brashness. They have a keen eye for beautiful things but are not overly materialistic. Harry agreed that these attributes were true of his personality.

Harry seemed to lack in confidence and as a result appeared dull and non-expressive. His bland facial expressions and monotonous tone of voice revealed his lack of aliveness and a deep-rooted sadness. When we brought this to Harry's attention he expressed that he often experienced bouts of depression. All of the above are fairly common traits for blue personality types.

Harry was uninterested in job promotions and even in spending time out with friends. Most of his evenings he spent at home on his own. Harry's challenge was to get on with life in a positive way instead of becoming submerged in a melancholic state.

Second position – GREEN

Green in the second position reflected Harry's wish to get out into wide open spaces. He loved the wild countryside and said that whenever he sat on top of a mountain, cliff, or hill-top, he experienced a deep state of freedom. It was clear that Harry gained tremendous pleasure and inner fulfilment from such introspective experiences. Then he expressed how much he wished he could spend more time outside. We suggested that he may be feeling trapped subconsciously, which he acknowledged. He wished he could leave his job as a computer operator. "Being cooped up in a stuffy office all day" was not his idea of how he wanted to spend the rest of his life. Harry wanted to use his creativity and express himself in a more meaningful way that would give him more inner satisfaction.

Third position – ORANGE

This color suggests that Harry should take a risk and go beyond his normal way of operating. By careful planning and taking constructive steps of action, Harry could begin the process of making moves toward fulfilling his innermost desires. Orange complements the blue in the first position. This means that his goals are in alignment with his true nature/ essence. This will help empower Harry to fulfill his true potential, bringing him joy and happiness and helping him to regain the inner spark and zest for life. We would recommend orange for Harry as the color most suited to his long-term needs, while he would require green color energy most whenever he felt trapped and caged in.

Action and advice

Before Harry could experience the energy of the color **orange** and use it productively, he needed to work with the **green** color energy for a while. We suggested that he should attend some Color Counselling sessions to help become more objective about his personal situation and help him achieve his goals and create what he really wanted in his life. Through his changing choices in the Color Reflection Reading in these sessions we could monitor his progress.

Harry really needed to work with his main challenge, reflected in his second position with the color **green.** Color Counselling sessions would help speed up the transition between **green** and **orange,** which would assist him to take whatever steps he felt were necessary to make real his aspirations in life. To date, Harry has received eight sessions over a four-month period. He no longer sees his situation at work as dull and dreary, but as a means to support him in his transition. His goal is stronger than ever and within the last four months he has been to the countryside hiking almost every second weekend. Harry is a much happier person and has begun to realize his own potential for creating his own reality.

THE LÜSCHER TEST   97

The Lüscher Test

The Lüscher color test is based on presenting a series of colored cards to a patient. Devised by Dr Max Lüscher, it has been used by psychologists and physicians since 1947. In the shortened version of the test, the practitioner asks you as the patient to place eight colors in order of preference. Your choices provide information about both your conscious and unconscious mind, your areas of stress, imbalances in your glandular system, and other physiological information. A trained practitioner can diagnose illness and, in some cases, forecast the outcome of an illness.

The basic colors of the test are the four "psychological primaries": blue, yellow, red, and green. The interpretation of the color choices is derived from the immediate physiological response, which is closely associated to deeper needs. Blue engenders calmness, while yellow (nearest to the color of natural light) brings activity. The brightness of yellow breaks down chemicals at the back of the eye – catabolism – while the darkness of blue allows rebuilding – anabolism. The same contrast is true of red and green; red breaks down and green rebuilds.

Your choice of a particular color depends on the extent to which your body needs anabolism or catabolism. If, for example, you are psychically or physically in need of emotional peace, physical regeneration, and release from tension or stress, then the instinctive response will be to choose darker colors. If you need to dissipate energy by mental or physical activity, your instinctive response will be toward brighter colors. In this way, the colors produce a sophisticated reading of your personality and needs.

Experienced color practitioners may feel ill at ease with the Lüscher Test. Color therapy takes into account the impact of the shape and form of the color being applied (see pp. 46-7). If you react in one way to the playing card shapes of the Lüscher Test, you could well react in a different way if they were all triangles, or diamond-shaped, for example. Some experimental tests confirm this.

The Lüscher Test is nonetheless a useful tool for investigating personality characteristics, though its healing application is limited.

Colors and their meaning

The significance of the eight colors in the shortened Lüscher Test depends on where they are placed in the scale of preference. When placed in the first, or "most preferred" position, their meanings closely resemble the meaning that color practitioners attach to them, as follows
Grey *Borderline, neutral, lack of commitment.*
Blue *Peace, tranquillity, calm.*
Green *Persistence, constancy, resistance to change.*
Red *Action, effectiveness, the "impact of the will".*
Yellow *Spontaneous enjoyment of action, uninhibited expansiveness, relaxation, release from burdens.*
Violet *Union of red and blue, wish fulfilment, intuitive understanding, sometimes irresponsibility, emotional immaturity.*
Brown *Contains red, but without red's vitality, strong sensation of bodily senses.*
Black *Extinction, negation.*

healing with color

Once you are familiar with the diagnostic methods described in Chapter Five, you can consult the chart on the facing page to see what forms of treatment to use. This chapter demonstrates and describes the tools and techniques of color therapy. It describes how a practitioner starts the healing process (see below), then presents the methods for color treatments. These fall into two main categories: those that use pigment color (see pp. 102-6) and those that use colored light (see pp. 108-22).

In the first category, using the color consciousness exercise (see pp. 103-6) helps to stimulate your memory, and your creative thinking. It can also help to heal paralysis following a stroke, and improve the nervous system, and eyesight. Using colored silks, clothes, and foods (see p. 105) gives you ways to back up a practitioner's treatments between sessions.

Colored light represents the most subtle, and therefore the most powerful, way to use color in healing. The most important development in color therapy has been the use of colored light equipment (see pp. 110-13), but there are other ways to harness the power of color. Color breathing and visualization techniques were described in Chapter Three; this chapter describes accessories to light treatments, from the color bath (see p. 114) that delivers colored light refracted through water, to the eye healing lamp (see p. 116), and the healing qualities of colored oils (see p. 117), and crystals (see pp. 117-18). The chapter also discusses how to combine methods of treatment, and how and when to bring treatment to a close (see p. 122). You can carry out most of the treatments for yourself at home, although the colored light treatments on pages 110-13 should only be carried out by a specialist color practitioner (see p. 111).

Receiving a patient

When a practitioner greets a patient, the first sensation on meeting comes from the emotions – the heart area, otherwise described as the soul. When you greet another person, you may not be aware of this level of the encounter; you probably allow your intellect to step in and make a mental appraisal of the person and the situation. Such an immediate appraisal often overrides the original intuitive experience of your own soul. The mental appraisal, which always follows the heart reaction, may justify your original feeling, but equally it might distort it by making an intellectual judgement that goes against your intuition. Trusting your immediate emotional response makes an important start to the healing process. It allows you to remain open to the messages that a person is giving you. The third part of your immediate experience is simply that of being confronted by another physical being (see pp. 44-5).

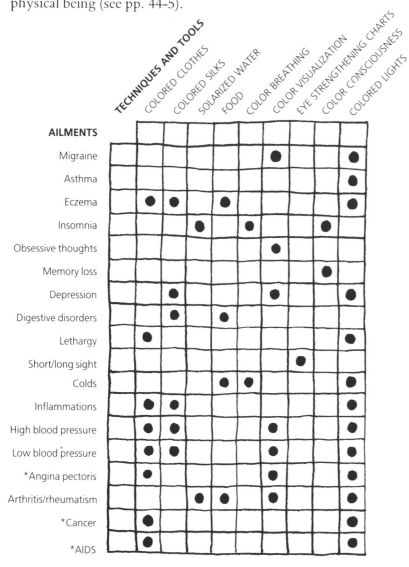

AILMENTS	COLORED CLOTHES	COLORED SILKS	SOLARIZED WATER	FOOD	COLOR BREATHING	COLOR VISUALIZATION	EYE STRENGTHENING CHARTS	COLOR CONSCIOUSNESS	COLORED LIGHTS
Migraine						●			●
Asthma									●
Eczema	●	●		●					●
Insomnia			●		●			●	
Obsessive thoughts						●			
Memory loss								●	
Depression		●				●			●
Digestive disorders		●		●					
Lethargy	●								●
Short/long sight							●		
Colds				●	●				●
Inflammations	●	●							●
High blood pressure	●	●				●			●
Low blood pressure	●	●				●			●
*Angina pectoris	●					●			●
Arthritis/rheumatism			●	●		●			●
*Cancer	●								●
*AIDS	●								●

*not to be treated without medical supervision

Underlying these three "confrontations" is the practitioner's meeting with the patient as a spiritual being manifest as a physical person. By acknowledging a patient at a spiritual level, and doing this first and foremost through the heart, and by trusting these feelings, the practitioner fully accepts the patient, and this is the first step toward treatment.

Spirituality and healing

Color therapy works on freeing the energy flow of the body. Fundamental to the healing process is the link between every person and a higher consciousness. This consciousness may be expressed as a universal power, God, or as a "oneness of being". The link can be called your "spirituality". The healing process requires the physical, emotional, and mental functions to work smoothly and in unison so that the energy of your body interchanges freely with the energy of the universe.

The practitioner, in the role of counsellor, talks to the patient (see pp. 84-5), and from this builds a picture of the most appropriate forms of treatment (see chart p. 101). The treatment may continue for several months, or be complete in one consultation (see p. 122). The practitioner may use a combination of several techniques, including giving the patient color exercises to do at home, in order to maintain the progress between treatment sessions with the practitioner.

Color consciousness exercise

This exercise presents color and shape in combination, thus engaging both the creative, right side and the logical, left side of the brain (see p. 46). The colors and forms are presented with their complementaries (see left). The first shape is the "container" and the second its "content" (see p. 47). These polarized energies increase your response to the image dramatically. The final card combines the two colors and shapes. Working toward integrating these challenges you on a mental, emotional, and physical level.

The exercise will improve your memory, your ingenuity, and your inventiveness. It also encourages creativity and artistic growth in children. As a healing technique, you can use the exercise to help insomnia, improve the nervous system, exercise the eyesight, and help in cases of paralysis after a stroke.

The exercise

To use the shapes, redraw the solid color to approximately 4.5ins (11cms) square, using paint or felt-tip pens. Place the first set of three cards on a wall 4-5 feet (1.2-1.5m) away from you. Fix your eyes on the first (container) shape for 15-30 seconds, then cover it with a blank white or grey sheet and relax your gaze on to this for 15-30 seconds. Then look at the centre of the second (content) shape for 15-30 seconds, cover it as before and look at the blank sheet. Finally, look at the third – the combination – image for the same time, and finish as before, by looking at the blank sheet.

Do this with the eight sets, morning and evening. A complete session lasts about 20 minutes. Repeat for 2-3 weeks.

Alternatively, use only two sets at a time. Choose complementary sets, for example, Set 1 (red) followed by Set 5 (turquoise). Allow yourself the freedom to choose the colors of the sets intuitively.

Natural daylight or full-spectrum lighting (see p. 36) supplies the best light for the exercise.

Container	Content	Combination

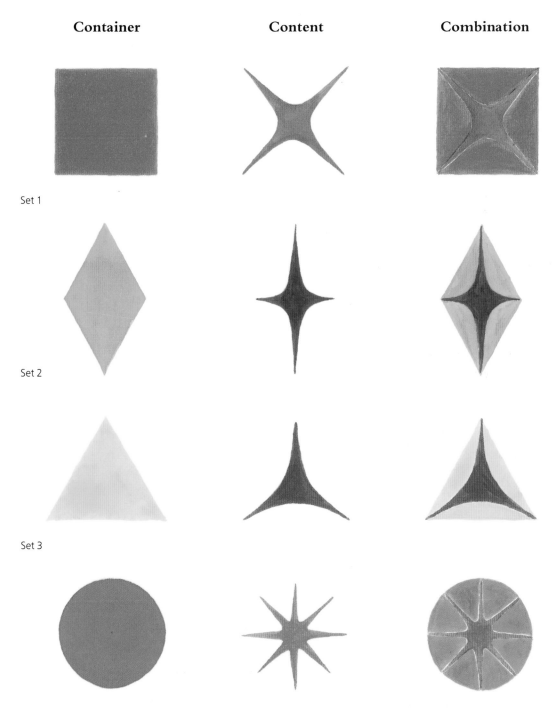

Set 1

Set 2

Set 3

Set 4

The Platonic Solids

Tetrahedron
(4 x 3)
Associated with fire, man, sight,
recognition, consciousness, and the
color red.

Octahedron
(8 x 3)
Associated with air, the bird, sound
(listening), pyramid healing energy,
and the color yellow.

Icosahedron
(20 x 3)
Associated with water, the reptile,
taste, and the color blue.

Hexahedron
(6 x 4)
Associated with earth, the mammal,
smell, and the color green.

Dodecahedron
(12 x 5)
Associated with ether, spirit, touch,
and the color violet.

Color, shape, and Sacred Geometry

Ancient geometry begins with the One, the basic Unity, the representation of the wholeness of the universe. The Ancient Greeks (7th-2nd centuries BC) produced geometric shapes to try to articulate all the spaces and relationships, patterns, and proportions existing within the original sphere of creation.
The shapes became known as the Sacred Geometry. Current Western scientific thinking now accepts the importance of patterns and proportional relationships between particles, and the notion that these (rather than the particles themselves) affect our perception.

Plato, a contemporary of the ancient geometricians, visualized the world as being composed of basic elements, each represented by a particular shape. Plato expressed them in five "Solids". The Platonic Solids are special versions of the Sacred Geometry. In each solid, the lengths of the sides are all equal, and all interior angles are equal. The elements are traditionally linked with color – fire being seen as red, water as blue, and so on.

The Platonic Solids represent a blueprint for all the cell structures in the bodies of humans, animals, plants, and minerals. The two-dimensional colored shapes used in healing are ultimately derived from the Platonic Solids.

The shapes based on triangles traditionally represent male energy; the hexahedron, built on the square, represents female energy. The dodecahedron, based on the pentagon, is the number of life (three male plus two female).

Working with colored pigment

Printed or dyed colors present a useful way of treating with color and maintaining progress between treatments with light. Some ailment treatments (see pp. 100, 102–3 and 107) are particularly suited to working with pigment color. The general effects of using color in interior decorating were discussed in Chapter One. The therapeutic use of these colors in clothes, silks, food, and the eye strengthening chart is described here.

When choosing colors, it is of course important to consider the appropriate shade. Try to find a tone that comes from the centre of the spectral color, not too dark or too light.

Colored clothes

The effects of wearing colored clothes follow the general patterns already described (see p. 22). For example, wear blue to reduce high blood pressure; red to give you more energy and to increase low blood pressure. Experience has shown that wearing red can cure infertility that results from low body temperature combined with low blood pressure. Wear orange to combat depression; turquoise to enhance your immunity and to help inflammatory conditions.

In all cases, it is advisable to wear natural fibres because they allow the body to breathe. This refers not only to the exchange of air, but to the exchange of the finer color energies in and out of the body.

Colored silks

Silk is the finest material for the transmission of color energies (see above). Allow yourself the luxury of using a large piece of silk to cover your undressed body, following the same color guide as above. Lie down, ideally with full daylight on your silk-covered body, and listen to your favourite music for about 20 minutes. Do this three times each week for maximum effect.

Food

The different colors of food appeal to the eye. You should trust your intuition, and take in the colors of food that you choose naturally. If you follow your own guidance, and are not beguiled by outside influences such as advertising, you will be choosing food colors that your body needs.

The value of pigment in treatment

From the theory that describes solid objects as light energy that has slowed down (see p. 37), it follows that the pigment in a solid object is also a form of light energy reduced into matter. Pigment contains a memory of the energy of the light from which it arose. Plants contain this memory, which is why plant dyes are thought to be more effective in healing than artificial ones. Pigment cannot penetrate the body in the way that light does, so its healing properties are less powerful than those of light.

Pigment and light

The distinction between the effectiveness of pigment and light in healing is not absolutely clear. The pigment in clothes and silks, for example, is effective because of the light that penetrates through the colored fabric and into the body.

The eye strengthening chart (see p. 106) produces a mixture of the effects of pigment and light. The eye fixes on the pigment color and turns it back into light by way of the after image.

Eye strengthening chart

Eye problems represent a deterioration of the processes that produce vision. Too much work that entails focusing at the same distance over extended periods impairs the function of the eyes. The eye strengthening chart (see left) can be used to re-activate tired eyes, or to re-stimulate the eyes on a daily basis to maintain healthy vision. For more serious problems, use the eye healing lamp described on page 116.

Healthy tissue undergoes a continual transformation, taking new material in, and shedding useless cells. The eye strengthening chart gently moves the energies and the cell structures, re-introducing a more lively activity. The blue expands the blood vessels, and relaxes the organism, while the red increases the level of activity. This expansion-contraction stimulates the whole eye.

Healing with light

Light and its colors come from the original energies of creation. Light energy can penetrate all living substances; it affects the biochemical structures of plants, animals, and human beings (see p. 20).

There are many ways of introducing light into the body. The color breathing and color visualization exercises in Chapter Three can be as powerful as any other sort of treatment. But the lamps used for color healing have a more direct influence. The color energies penetrate your body and this does not depend on your ability to visualize.

Using the eye strengthening chart

Focus your eyes first on the blue octagonal shape. Maintain your gaze for 15-20 seconds. Then look at a blank sheet of white or grey paper for 15-20 seconds. The after image will appear, and then fade. Now look at the red shape, and repeat the exercise. Continue in this way, six times daily.

You can reproduce this chart for yourself or obtain a printed copy (see Resources, p. 124) and place it on a wall at eye level where you have access to it daily.

Container	Content	Combination

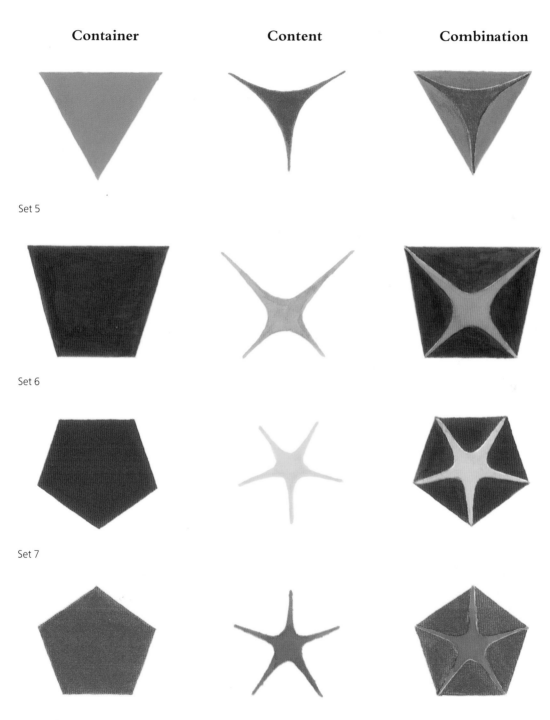

Set 5

Set 6

Set 7

Set 8

This section (pp. 108-23) deals with the techniques of using the healing qualities of colored light. It describes first the use of colored lamps (pp. 108-13), one of the main healing sources in color therapy. It then goes on to discuss other accessories available to practitioners, such as the eye healing lamp (p. 116) and the Hy-Co-Jet bath (p. 114). The final sections describe techniques you can use at home, such as solarized water (p. 115), and the use of oils (p. 117) and crystals (pp. 117-8).

Color therapy instruments

Equipment for projecting colored light on to a patient can be designed in various ways, but the first instrument to combine color and form for this purpose was designed at Hygeia Studios in Gloucestershire, England, in 1969.

The color therapy instrument uses a full-spectrum lamp housed in a box. One side of the box is designed to take a piece of frosted glass, a stained glass filter, and lastly a screen, or "mask", which controls the shape of the light aperture. In this way, the treatment color can be combined with the particular shape that enhances its work (see p. 47). The shapes correspond to those already seen in the color consciousness exercise (see pp. 102-3 and p. 107).

The high quality of the stained glass filter ensures that the full spectrum of the required color is projected on to the patient. The filters are made by hand, but their chemical composition resembles the structure of the natural oxides found in jewels. Gold, silver, copper, magnesium, and cobalt are incorporated into liquid quartz, then mouth blown and cut into sheets.

Light treatment

Once the treatment color has been determined, whether through spinal diagnosis, or aura analysis, or any of the other diagnostic techniques described in Chapter Five, the practitioner may decide to treat with colored light using the color therapy instrument.

Exposure to the treatment color alternates with its complementary. The treatment color orange alternates with blue; magenta with green; violet with yellow, and red with turquoise. The patient prepares for treatment by stepping into an all-white gown, so as not to distort the colors that penetrate through clothing to the body, and then sits or lies down in comfort about 6–8 feet (2m) from the color therapy instrument. The two colors are set on a stand, the treatment color above the complementary color (see below).

In addition to combining color and shape, the light treatment is delivered in a rhythmic way. The timing of these exposures is operated by a time control and is based on the proportions of the "golden mean" (see p. 38). The initial exposure to the treatment color is ¾ minute, then the instrument switches to the complementary for 3¼ minutes. As the exposure to the treatment color increases to 5¼ minutes, the length of the exposure to the complementary decreases to ¾ minute (see below). The total exposure time is 19¾ minutes, of which the treatment color accounts for 12½ minutes, and the complementary 7¼ minutes, thus keeping to the "golden mean" proportions. An example of the times of exposure to a color and its complementary is given below, shown in quarters of a minute.

The need for the complementary color

Experience has shown that treatment with one color only does not produce a healing result. It may improve the symptoms, which then revert to the pretreatment condition on exposure to daylight. Research into treatment for high blood pressure has indicated that this is the case.

As all energy exists with its complementary energy, the use of the complementary color in therapy makes a natural pattern for treatment.

Treatment times for colored light

Treatment color	orange	3/4	5/4	8/4	13/4	21/4	minutes
Complementary color	blue	13/4	8/4	5/4	3/4		minutes

The color therapy instrument

This instrument (left), *developed by the Hygeia Studios, provides full-spectrum color defined in the shape that enhances that color's effect* (see pp. 110–11). *The exposure to the treatment color* (top) *and its complementary* (bottom) *is rhythmic and carefully timed* (see above).

The instrument is used in a darkened room to prevent daylight "diluting" the effects of the colors used in treatment.

At the end of each phase of color, one light is dimmed gradually while at the same time the other is slowly turned up to full strength. The patient may have relaxed into sleep, which is a good sign, because this ensures that the colors are well absorbed.

After the treatment, or as the patient awakes, there might be an immediate emotional response, resulting from the release of blocked emotional energies. This can have an immediate effect on the colors of the aura. Grey discolorations, representing unaccepted energy may have been absorbed, and brown areas, the result of energy not being let go, may have lessened, or disappeared (see p. 89). The colors may generally have become brighter and clearer. Such changes may be "momentary" (24-72 hours), "temporary" (2-12 weeks), or permanent.

The treatment colors

MAGENTA
The key to magenta is the idea of *letting go*. Use it also where change is needed. Magenta induces spirituality – it brings with it a recognition of spiritual energies.

VIOLET
The keyword for using violet is *dignity*.

BLUE
The keyword for blue is *relaxation*.

TURQUOISE
The theme for the work of turquoise is *immunity*.

Mental
Use magenta if you need to let go of old thought patterns, or old memories.

Mental
Violet works on your feelings of self worth, your dignity, and your self respect. Use it if you tend to diminish yourself, and always feel that others can do better than you.

Mental
Use blue when you cannot think calmly, or when you have no patience with your thoughts; when you always feel determined you are hurrying.

Mental
Use turquoise when you are dominated by others; when you do not rely on your own thoughts, but throw them away and value other people's ideas more. In other words, use it when you lack immunity to other people's thoughts.

The safety of light treatments

Before starting color therapy treatments it is wise to consult a trained practitioner. However, the treatments using colored silk, clothes, and food can be used at home. If you select and use the wrong treatment color, although you will not gain any benefit from the treatment, you will not do any lasting damage.

Treatments using colored light are more powerful. It is important that the treatments given with the color healing instruments described on pages 108-17 are only given by people trained in the use of the instrument. The correct timing of the light exposure is as critical as the selection of the correct color for treatment. The wrong rhythm can create imbalances in the body's energy flow, and correcting these imbalances may require further treatment.

GREEN
The keyword for green is *balance.*

YELLOW
The central theme for yellow is *detachment.*

ORANGE
The keyword for orange is *joy.*

RED
The keyword for red is *energy.*

Mental
Use green if you tend to take your work home with you, in the metaphorical sense; equally, when you take your domestic matters into your work situation. Use it if you cannot keep your thoughts in balance; if they are dominated by one thing or another.

Mental
When you cannot detach yourself from other people's activity; you cannot make your own thoughts, or you become over-attached to an idea that you need to let go of, consider using yellow.

Mental
If you cannot enjoy your own mental processes, or just do not feel like using your brain to do anything, use orange.

Mental
If you lack mental energy even to think, and you do not want to get involved with anything, use red.

MAGENTA

Emotional
When old feelings no longer apply, magenta works on these unwanted emotions, allowing you freedom to let go of them and to grow and change.

Metabolic
For problems within the home; use magenta when you need to let go of old domestic patterns and make changes in the rhythm or conduct of the household, including meal times and any domestic routines.

Physical
This level affects the plan of the day or week. Use magenta if you need to set aside existing schedules and restructure the daily or weekly plan.

VIOLET

Emotional
If you do not like your own feelings, or think they are of no interest, use violet. It is the color most deeply associated with your feelings about who you really are.

Metabolic
Use violet if you lack respect for your home, or do not treat it in a dignified way. Violet is indicated when your home is just a place you use, rather than live in fully.

Physical
This refers to lack of self love, or lack of self appreciation. Use violet if you feel that you are not beautiful.

BLUE

Emotional
If you cannot experience peaceful feelings, or feel ill at ease with your feelings, consider using blue.

Metabolic
When you have no time for your home, your food, or your lifestyle, or if you are the type who snatches a quick sandwich in one hand and has a book in the other at the same time, you need blue treatment.

Physical
Try using blue when everything is rushed, when you never seem to have enough time for your daily tasks or your weekly schedule.

TURQUOISE

Emotional
When you find you are laughing with other people, even when you do not understand what is funny, consider using turquoise. You may also find that other people's illnesses affect you; they make you feel ill, too.

Metabolic
Turquoise works on the immunity of the cell. Use it when your health immunity is low, and you too readily catch infections.

Physical
The habit of imitating others, or "keeping up with the neighbours", suggests the need for the color turquoise. Use it when you cannot help being influenced by other people's style of living.

GREEN

Emotional
When you feel unbalanced by relationships that are no longer intact, treat with green.

Metabolic
Green induces balance in the household and in the body. Use it when your home or your health is unbalanced.

Physical
If your daily programme is unbalanced – you do not eat breakfast, or you skip lunch – or if you have the feeling that you cannot get things sorted out, think of using green in your healing.

YELLOW

Emotional
For people who cannot stand back from a situation; for a mother who rushes to her baby immediately at the merest sound, yellow is helpful.

Metabolic
This relates to the calcium uptake process in the body. Calcium accumulates at the joints through an inability to let it go. People over 40 years old may need yellow.

Physical
Use yellow to enable you to detach yourself from your material possessions – your old car, or curtains that you may have had for a long time and can no longer use, but feel unable to relinquish.

ORANGE

Emotional
Lack of joy or happiness in a relationship often goes unmentioned, but if you do not enjoy your emotional experiences you will need more of this color. It is used to combat depression. If you overdo treatment with orange, the opposite feelings can set in: you become happy-go-lucky and irresponsible.

Metabolic
If your home circumstances do not give you joy, if you no longer enjoy meal times, or if you feel no joy when preparing food, treat with orange.

Physical
Treat unhappiness that permeates all your activities – a general lethargy, or a feeling that you can't be bothered with things – with orange. Endless procrastination suggests that you need orange.

RED

Emotional
You have not even enough energy to experience any emotions, or your emotions lack strength. You are too tired to bother with your emotions. All these symptoms suggest that you need red.

Metabolic
Use red if no energy is being put into the household; if everything is being done for convenience and not for the pleasure of doing it. If, for example, you are too tired to lay the table attractively before eating, or you rely on artificial room fresheners or any other prop to reduce the amount of effort needed in the house, try red.

Physical
Use red to counter physical apathy. It also raises blood pressure; it treats low blood pressure.

Colored oils (right), *for massage or in baths, can be used to complement color therapy treatments. Ideally the oils should be used freshly made (see p. 117).*

Color healing accessories

You can use the range of color healing accessories discussed in this section either in combination with the color therapy instrument, or as healing tools in themselves. Refer to the chart on page 101 to see which ailments respond best to which treatment.

Hy-Co-Jet bath

By exposing yourself to colored light in water, you can absorb the light frequencies over the whole surface of your body. The warmth of the water, combined with the massage from the jets at the sides of the bath, relaxes your muscles and makes your body more receptive to color.

The Hy-Co-Jet bath may be fitted with any color, but usually it is used with blue and its complementary, orange, to reduce stress, insomnia, and muscle tension. Fill the bath with water that is comfortably hot, and once you are in, switch on the jets alone for up to five minutes before starting the color treatment. At this point, stop the jets, and enjoy the colors. The start button sets in motion a time control: the same timings apply as with the color therapy instrument (see p. 109), so the colored bath session ends after

The Hy-Co-Jet bath
Jets of water from the sides of the bath relax the patient before the light treatment begins. An automatic time control mechanism controls the exposure to the treatment color and its complementary.

19¾ minutes. At this point the temperature of the water will have cooled slightly, to blood heat. Getting out at this point presents the least shock to the system. Play some soothing music during your bath to enhance the effects (see p. 118).

Water solarizer

The colors of light are thought to affect water at the molecular level, imbuing the water with the energies of the color that it receives, as well as affecting its taste. Solarized water was used in Ayurvedic medicine in India from the 1st century AD, but it may have been first made there as long as 9000 years ago. It was also used for healing in Egypt about 4000 years ago.

To solarize water, surround a glass of still water with a full-spectrum filter of red or blue (see *Resources,* p. 124). Allow sunlight to shine through the glass for about two hours (longer on a cloudy day). Then drink the water slowly.

The taste changes according to the color of the filter: red makes the water sour; blue sweetens it. Other colors produce a range of tastes between these two extremes. For this reason, only red and blue are usually used. Use the red filter as a stimulation – to help you wake up, for example. The blue solarized water has a relaxing effect, and is a good bedtime drink.

Eye healing lamp

Use the eye healing lamp for severe disturbances of the eye, such as cataracts, and glaucoma. It also improves short and long sight, by mobilizing the muscles of the iris, which control the shape of the lens.

The lamp has one color aperture and two filters. Sit about three feet (0.7-0.9m) in front of the lamp, with the aperture at eye level. Move the turquoise and red filters over the aperture in turn, so that you see first the turquoise colored light, then the red. Look at each color for 20-30 seconds. Gaze at the white, black, or grey panel at the base of the lamp for 20-30 seconds between each color; this allows the eye to produce the after-image color (see p. 62), which relaxes the eye. Do this twice daily. Finish with the turquoise, and its after image, so that the eyes are completely relaxed at the end of the session. Consult your eye specialist to monitor the effects of the lamp.

Eye healing lamp and Cocrysto
The eye healing lamp (left) and Cocrysto (right) have been developed at the Hygeia Studios, Gloucestershire, England.

The eye healing lamp is about 13ins (33cm) tall. Stand it on a table and sit in front of it, using the red and turquoise filters according to the instructions given on page 116.

The Cocrysto is a hand-held torch that uses the healing energies of crystals, programmed with the healing color by a stained glass filter (see below) to bring color energy into the chakras.

Oils
Colored oils are made from pure oils by the addition of healing herbs and flowers and exposure to sunlight, often for days or weeks. This allows the oils to absorb the energy of the plants; the oil also changes color, depending on which plant is used.

Use the oils to massage part or all of the body or in a bath. The particular energies of each oil may be soothing or ener-gizing in their effects, depending on the plants used. Ideally, fresh oils should be used and always remember to follow the manufacturer's instructions.

Crystals
Crystals are concentrated forms of light energy that are produced in the absolute darkness of coal beds, clay beds, and other sedimentary rocks. Because of their structure, they can absorb instructions via the electronic messages from a computer. Using light and a colored filter, a quartz crystal can be programmed for healing with that color.

In the same way as the chakras are seen as being the energy centres of the human body, so the crystals are the energy centres of our planet Earth. By using crystals in healing, you will be able to tune your body to the healing energy of the planet.

In the same way as the chakras are seen as being the energy centres of the human body, so the crystals are the energy centres of our planet (see right). By using crystals in healing, you can tune the body to the healing energy of the planet.

Enhancing therapy with music

Music may be used as part of the treatment plan. It can be a powerful support to the work of color treatment, in three ways.

First, background music can be used for its healing qualities. The composer JS Bach incorporated intervals into his music that bore the same relationship to each other as numbers in the Fibonacci series (see p. 38). These musical intervals create, in effect, the same "golden mean" proportions that are seen in classical architecture, and that are said to create a visual harmony. In the same way, music produces a vibratory harmony – healing sounds.

Second, musically qualified practitioners can develop personalized musical themes that stimulate the memory and the subconscious of the individual.

Third, the practitioner may encourage you to sing. This both helps you to express yourself freely, and to "retune" your body, by linking your mind, your body, and your emotions. The following three case studies indicate how a practitioner interprets patients' problems and demonstrates the way a course of color therapy can progress.

Crystals are used in color therapy to balance the chakra system of a patient (see p. 64). Clear and colorless quartz crystals are the most useful in color healing. The color crystal torch, or Cocrysto (see p. 117), focuses light through a stained glass filter and a clear quartz crystal to bring color into the chakras. The patient should be dressed in white, as colored clothing will distort the treatment color. Hold the Cocrysto about one inch (2.5cm) from the patient's body, focusing the energies through visualization on to each chakra centre.

Combining treatments

Ideally all color therapy should be supervised by a qualified practitioner. By getting to know the patient, the practitioner can use his or her professional judgement about how often to treat, and how many therapeutic methods to combine. It is quite usual to use two methods to maximize the effect. A practitioner will usually give a patient color breathing exercises (see p. 54) or guided visualizations (see p. 52) that back up the work of the color therapy instrument. Alternatively, the patient may receive advice on colored clothing (see p. 105) to wear to maintain the effects. Treatments support each other best when identical colors are used.

Consult the chart on page 101 to see which ailments respond well to two or more methods used in combination. To a large extent, the choice of treatments is a practical solution to a particular problem. For example, it would be of little use to suggest a visualization to treat insomnia, as the images would be more likely to keep the patient awake than to induce sleep. Instead, if you are being treated for insomnia with the color therapy instrument, you might choose to drink blue solarized water between treatments. You could also add color breathing. If so, give yourself a break – ideally overnight – between drinking the solarized water and using the breathing techniques. This break allows your body to absorb the energy of the treatments.

Increasing the number of techniques or the exposure to color does not necessarily speed the healing process. Too much color cannot be absorbed by the body; you can "overdose" on color just as you can on drugs. As a general rule, do not exceed one treatment in every 24 hours.

The following three case studies indicate how a practitioner interprets patients' problems and demonstrates the way a course of color therapy can progress.

Case study – Trevor

Trevor's case was interesting because it showed very clearly that he was blocking some unhappy thoughts about his life. Following an operation for cancer, he was depressed and aimless. Aged 62, he was not looking forward to retirement.

He resented the fact that his wife worked long hours. Generally it was difficult to get him to talk about himself. Even when I asked about his hobbies, he said that his interest in woodwork had gone since he found it painful to get involved in an activity that was associated with the period before his illness.

Advice and treatment

The color that came up from the spinal diagnosis was orange, specifically relating to the emotional area. One way to approach his problem of depression and his lack of ability to talk about himself was to get him involved in an activity that confronted his emotions. I encouraged him to take up woodwork again.

The color yellow came up in the metabolic area at the next treatment. I asked him to work on a visualization to help him detach from painful memories of the past. I felt that the significance of his metabolic problem may be deep-seated, or too problematic to treat. Sometimes it can be more effective to tackle the problem via another avenue, as in the visualization. The operative factor was the color, yellow, which gave the clue that detachment was needed.

After five treatments, Trevor's problems seemed to lift considerably, through working obliquely to encourage him to create change and acknowledge the areas of his life that he was blocking from his consciousness.

Case study – Natasha

Natasha came to me with a persistent problem of general weakness and tiredness. She felt unable to "get the day started". We talked about her life and I questioned her about her domestic life and her work. I wanted to know which of her activities she most enjoyed, and which of them she found unpleasant. After a long discussion it became clear that my client looked forward to nothing at all.

We talked about her eating habits, which are a key factor in the health of the metabolic activity in the body. "I usually eat anything that doesn't need to be prepared", she said. "Often I buy a sandwich or something that I can heat up quickly." Natasha lived alone, and had little opportunity for joining friends or family for lunch or dinner.

She was equally scathing about how she spent her spare time. Natasha wanted to write, but felt she had no chance of learning how to begin.

Advice and treatment

Natasha was obviously not getting enough nutrition from her food. This seemed to be more overriding than her frustrated ambition to write. Her spinal diagnosis showed the need for treatment with the color green.

I treated her with this using the color therapy instrument.

I continued the treatments over the next few weeks, following up problems with Natasha's digestion, by setting exercises for her to carry out at home. Turquoise showed up as the treatment color at the second consultation. I gave her some turquoise paper, which she was to place over her abdomen, and use to enable her to practise color breathing, taking turquoise in and breathing red out.

By incorporating fresh fruit and vegetables into her diet, and after the color breathing, there were improvements in Natasha's digestion and in her energy level. She could now address her wish to write, and sounded much more clear about it. She continued color breathing, taking turquoise in, and breathing red out.

When, at the next session, orange came up as a treatment color, it was time to concentrate on her own fulfilment – to try writing, and to use this to bring more joy into her life. She seemed ready to begin. Before the next treatment, Natasha started writing. But she stopped her color breathing, and this showed up in her reduced energy levels. Once Natasha understood that her own work was just as important as the therapy sessions, she started the exercises again. The successful outcome of the treatment was the publication of her first book a year later.

Case study – Melanie

I first met Melanie when she was nine years old. She did not speak or allow any eye contact. As soon as she saw me, she ran out of the house and raced around the garden on her bicycle.

Her father and mother told me that when she was two months old, Melanie had had an operation to remove a facial mark. After the operation, her mother noticed a change in Melanie, "It was as if I lost contact completely, I cannot describe it any other way." Her father enlarged on this, "The doctors admitted that it had been very difficult to bring Melanie round after the operation."

I realized that the shock of the operation had been too great for Melanie at that early age. The operation had shifted her protective aura away from her body (see pp. 88-9) and it had not returned to normal. The mental and emotional areas were not connecting with the metabolic and physical areas. Melanie seemed to hover above her body, unable to "connect" with it.

Both parents agreed that I should try to treat her. I knew that it would take many months, but they agreed to be patient.

Advice and treatment

For a whole year I treated Melanie, seeing her every three to four weeks. One day, her spinal diagnosis chart looked completely different from all previous ones. When I met Melanie again, she looked straight into my eyes.

Melanie continued to make eye contact during the next few months. By this time, I had made 26 spinal diagnosis charts. None of the active vertebrae in the emotional area of the early charts were paired, and there was no connection between the mental/ emotional and the physical/ metabolic areas. But by now, Melanie was producing more and more normal charts. After about three years of work, she began to speak. Her parents were delighted.

Today, when I meet Melanie, she seems very obviously a "normal" child. Anyone who met her without knowing her history would never suspect anything was wrong.

Melanie still dislikes reading, and, indeed, cannot, as yet, read fluently, nor does she like writing. But this is not surprising after such a history. A great deal of care and more patience has to be given to her. But in general, she is now a very happy, peaceful, and healthy young lady.

As the sun sets the colors of the evening do not fade into the colors of the night, but are still present at the deeper level of the invisible (right).

Finishing the healing process

Treatments with a practitioner might continue over a few weeks or a few months. A review of progress takes place at regular intervals. This gives both the patient and the practitioner the opportunity to reflect on the changes and to see how well the patient is responding to self treatment at home. Repeated color diagnosis via the aura or using the spinal diagnosis, or the Color Reflection Reading (see pp. 94-6), monitors these changes.

Before a patient stops treatment, the practitioner looks again at the patient's understanding of the connection between mind, body, and emotions (see p. 74). The key feature of healing is to accept the role of the emotions. If the emotional response, which is the first response, is not acknowledged, these stifled feelings begin to create problems in the mind and body. By encouraging the patient to feel involved with the emotions, not to be ashamed of them or frightened by them, the practitioner ensures that the patient enriches his or her life within. By acknowledging, too, the role of rhythm, at work, at home, and in eating habits, the patient will be taking care of the metabolic aspect of health. Rhythm is not the same as meaningless routine: it simply addresses the need for regularity, but also regular change. It is a way of acknowledging daily the role of complementary energies that keep us in health.

A patient who has received treatment from a color therapist will not just feel better. Color therapy introduces a new way of looking at color, and because of this it can permanently enhance color awareness. Color becomes a new language for interpreting feelings, and recognizing the feelings of other people. It reconnects you to the rhythmic color energies of the planet, and enhances the living qualities of all life forms. The subtle powers of color that permeate you and all life will continually revitalize you.

BIBLIOGRAPHY

Gimbel, Theo. *The Color Therapy Workbook.* Element Books, Inc., 1993.

Gimbel, Theo. *Healing Through Colour.* Beekman Publishers, Inc. 1993.

Brennan, Barbara Ann. *Light Emerging:* The Journey of Personal Healing. Bantam Books, New York, 1993.

Gimbel, Theo. & Wills, Pauline. *Sixteen Steps to Health & Energy:* A Program of Color & Visual Meditation. Movement & Chakra Balance. Llewellyn Publication, Minnesota, 1992.

Wills, Pauline & Gimbel, Theo. *The Transformation Workbook:* Colour Healing & Yoga. Trans-Atlantic Publications, Inc., W. Foulsham, UK, 1992.

Babbitt, Edwin D. *Principles of Light and Color.* Sun Publishing, New Mexico, 1992.

Wood, Betty. *The Healing Power of Color:* How to Use Color to Improve Your Mental, Physical and Spiritual Well-Being. Destiny Books, Vermont, 1992.

Lieberman, Dr. Jacob. *Light: Medicine of the Future:* How We Can Use it to Heal Ourselves NOW. Bear & Co., New Mexico, 1991.

Latimer, Jane E. *Healing Power of Inner Light-Fire:* Accessing Higher Consciousness to Heal Your Life. LivingQuest, 1990.

Brennan, Barbara Ann. *Hands of Light:* A Guide to Healing Through the Human Energy Field, Bantam Books, New York, 1988.

Birren, Faber. *Symbolism of Color:* The Beauty and Magic of Color Has Been a Vital Part of Living, Religion, and Mysticism. Carol Publishing, 1988.

Ott, John. *Health & Light.* Devin, Connecticut, 1988.

Clark, Linda & Martine, Yvonne. *Health, Youth and Beauty Through Color Breathing.* Celestial Arts, California, 1976.

Clark, Linda. *Color Therapy.* Devin, Connecticut, 1975.

RESOURCES
Associations, Institutes, and Societies

The International Association for Color Therapy
73 Elm Bank Gardens
London SW13 0NX
Phone 011-44-0453-832150

California Institute for Integral Studies
San Francisco, CA
Phone 415-753-6100

Manifesting Inner Light
Sausalito, CA
Phone 415-332-4663

Omega Institute for Holistic Studies
260 Lake Drive
Rhinebeck, NY 12572
Phone 914-266-4301

Barbara Brennan School of Healing
P.O. Box 2005
East Hampton, NY 11937
Phone 516-324-9745
Fax 516-324-9745
(lectures, workshops, and 4-Year Professional Healing Science Training Program)

New York Open Center
A Nonprofit Holistic Learning Center
83 Spring Street
New York, NY 10012
Phone 212-219-2527
Fax 212-219-1347

EQUIPMENT

Full Spectrum Lighting
Unit 1,
Riverside Business Centre
Victoria Street
High Wycombe
Bucks HP11 2LT
England

True-Lite Full Spectrum Fluorescent Lighting; SAD Portable Lightboxes

Hygeia Manufacturing Ltd
Hygeia Studios
Brook House, Avening
Glos GL8 8NS
England

Colour Space Illuminator; Pure Light Lamp; Crystal Lamp; Eye Healing Lamp; Hygeia Colour Wall; Hygeia Colour Therapy Instrument

Pool Services Ltd
Unit 12-14 Woodside Park Industrial Estate
Catteshall Lane
Godalming, Surrey GU7 1LG
England

Hy-Co-Jet Hydro Colour Therapy Jet Bath

AUTHOR'S ACKNOWLEDGEMENTS

I would like to extend my very special thanks to my wife Honor, who has offered objective opinions on the writing of this book. My thanks go also to Pauline Wills, tutor-in-charge at the Hygeia College of Colour Therapy, who gave practical advice on my writing and to Eleanor Lines at Gaia, who advised me on the content of the book. My staff, Doreen Cox and Rita Legg, have been very supportive, despite my occasional bouts of disgruntledness. Lastly, I should like to acknowledge the inspiration I have received from Father Dr Andrew Glazewski and Sir George Trevelyan, who have given me insight into the spiritual meaning of healing.

PUBLISHER'S ACKNOWLEDGEMENTS

Gaia Books Ltd would like to thank Rachel Adams, Suzy Boston, Ursula Browning, Gill Cormode, Fritz Fuchs, Natasha Goddard, Stuart Hall, Pamela Jenkins, Kate McNulty, Philip Parker, Kitty Parker-Jervis, Lesley Parry, Katherine Pate, Sonya Richards, Robert Rose, Howard Sun, Susan Walby, and Nan Wise for editorial and production work; Mary Warren for editorial assistance and the index; Select Typesetters; Global Colour, Malaysia.

PHOTOGRAPHIC CREDITS

pp, 2-3, 11, 14, 23, 42, 51, 55, 58, 78, 87, 98, 123, **Comstock;** p. 6 Manfred Cage/**Science Photo Library;** p. 19 **Sonia Halliday Photographs;** p. 27 Hugh Palmer/**IPC Magazines Ltd. 1989, Robert Harding Syndication;** p. 30 David Parker/**Science Photo Library;** p. 35 Fred Burrell/**Science Photo Library;** p. 38 **Paul Brierley Photos;** p. 75 Lynne Brotchie/ **The Garden Picture Library;** p. 115 Philip Dowell/**Gaia Books;** p. 119 Roberto du Gugliemo/ **Science Photo Library.**

index

Bold type indicates main entry